Herpes: The Facts

Dr J. K. Oates qualified in medicine at the London Hospital
Medical College in 1946. Following national service with the
Royal Air Force in the Middle East, he commenced an initial
spell of training as a pathologist at the London Hospital. Shortly
after this, he began to work in the field of sexually transmitted
diseases at the same hospital, spending time at the Johns
Hopkins Hospital in Baltimore and then as a research fellow
with the Medical Research Council.

For the last twenty-three years he has been the Physician in
Charge of the Departments of Genito-Urinary Medicine at
Addenbrooke's Hospital, Cambridge, and the Westminster
Hospital, London. He is the author of a number of papers on a
variety of aspects of his special subject and greatly enjoys
teaching anyone who will listen to him. Herpes has interested
him since the age of eleven, when he first contracted the lip
herpes from which he still suffers regularly and with stoicism.

J. K. OATES

Herpes: The Facts

PENGUIN BOOKS

Penguin Books Ltd, Harmondsworth, Middlesex, England
Penguin Books, 625 Madison Avenue, New York, New York 10022, U.S.A.
Penguin Books Australia Ltd, Ringwood, Victoria, Australia
Penguin Books Canada Ltd, 2801 John Street, Markham, Ontario, Canada L3R 1B4
Penguin Books (N.Z.) Ltd, 182–190 Wairau Road, Auckland 10, New Zealand

First published 1983

Made and printed in Great Britain by
Richard Clay (The Chaucer Press) Ltd, Bungay, Suffolk
Set in Photina

Contents

Acknowledgements

My thanks are due to the Departments of Medical Illustration and Photography at Addenbrooke's and the Westminster Hospitals for help with the illustrations, to Professor R. W. Horne of the Department of Ultrastructural Studies, the John Innes Institute, Norwich, for the diagram of a herpes virus capsid and to my colleagues and their technical staff in the departments of microbiology in my two hospitals for much help and advice. A special note of thanks is due to Dr Jack Nagington of the Public Health Laboratory Service Cambridge, who has taught me much about herpes simplex virus and its machinations over the past few years. I would hasten to add that any inaccuracies and all opinions expressed in the book are mine alone!

Finally, I would like to thank my secretaries Mary Mashiter and Pam Whitty for their invaluable help with so many things and Gloria Loom for typing the final manuscript.

*

The illustration on page 26 is from The Institute of Biology's Studies in Biology No. 95, *The Structure and Function of Viruses* by Robert W. Horne, published by Edward Arnold, London.

Introduction

Twenty years ago, I wrote a number of leaflets concerning the common sexually transmitted diseases. My reason for doing this was that patients were often so worried about what they feared was wrong with them that they did not understand, or even listen very closely, when they were told what was wrong. Also I had to admit that sometimes they did not get all the explanation that they should have done.

All the usual illnesses were covered, but when my colleagues and I got to herpes we could only write about eight lines, and a debate ensued as to whether it was worth printing such a short account. We did print it, but it was rather a pathetic and little-used leaflet. Some eight years later, when we re-wrote the series, we had no problem in writing twenty or so lines on herpes. By that time there was more to say about it and more need for information.

In 1980, so many people were asking about herpes that I wrote a twelve-page booklet on the subject, designed especially for those who were worried about the disease. It wasn't enough – the booklet answered many questions and relieved many anxieties, but it also posed additional and more complex questions. It also made it clear that very many people were worried about genital herpes.

That is the reason for this book, which is an attempt to explain to patients what I know about this illness and, above all, to try to put the disorder into some sort of perspective. It has caused, and still causes, many of my patients more anxiety and unhappiness than any other disease that I treat, and in my opinion much of this load of worry is, in the majority of cases, quite unnecessary.

There remains, however, a core of sufferers for whom genital herpes is a major problem, and they require all the sympathy and help the profession of medicine can offer. I hope that some of the information in this book will at least help to dispel some anxieties and misconceptions.

I have not found it an easy book to write, as I have been conscious that, while many readers will know little of the intricacies of modern biology, virology and so forth, others will be professionals and know very much more than I do. To attempt to do justice to the two sides and make the book both readable and reasonably accurate has inevitably led to some compromises being made.

CHAPTER 1
The History of a Disease

The subject of this book is a virus – herpes simplex virus – and how it coexists with man, occasionally causing him disease. In some ways it is a biography – a story of the virus's life – and, like all good biographies, it will take a close look at the family background and pay special attention to its nearest relations in that family. Where the virus lives and how it breeds, its whole life-style, will come under scrutiny. Our interest in this little bundle of nucleic acid lies in the fact that the virus's home is us – it takes up residence in us and stays with us as long as we are a functioning, live, biological unit. While with us, it tries relentlessly to send some of its progeny on to find another host – in short to infect another person. During our lives we and the virus may come into conflict from time to time – very, very infrequently when we consider the fact that by middle age virtually the whole of that population will be playing host to herpes simplex. These infrequent episodes of conflict represent herpetic disease, and we shall look into the various factors which in many Western cultures have led to one special form of the disease, namely genital herpes, becoming much more of a problem than was formerly the case.

Early History

We shall start with a look at the history of the illness and its name. Straight away, two important points can be very firmly made: firstly, herpes is in no way new and, secondly, when christened, its names were not very well chosen.

Herpes is certainly a very old disease; indeed some think it is one of our oldest viral diseases, and it may have been with us since the Pleistocene era, over a million years ago. One of the earliest references in medical texts is that attributed to the Greek physician Hippocrates, who gave an account of ulceration of the lips in 'intermittent fevers'. From this description it is clear that it is herpes of the lip, 'herpes labalis', the common fever blisters or cold sores, which are being described and that the physicians of the day were thoroughly familiar with them.

The name 'herpes' leads us into difficulties the moment we begin to try to trace some of the illness's history. The Greeks didn't give these sores the name of 'herpes', though the word is a Greek one meaning 'to creep' or 'to move like a serpent'. They, and other doctors after them, used the word to describe a host of very different illnesses, most of them involving the skin and sharing only a common tendency to spread locally or 'creep'. Fungus infection (ringworm), erysipelas (a streptococcal skin infection), cancer of the skin and a number of other illnesses all bear the title of 'herpes' in these ancient texts. Interestingly, one of the skin illnesses was well named. This was the common 'shingles', or 'herpes zoster' to give it its official name, and this is actually due to infection with another herpes virus, 'varicella zoster'.

The consequence of this widespread use of the word 'herpes' for so many different conditions is that it makes the task of tracing the printed history of the disorder so much more difficult unless the author writing about the illness gives such a clear-cut description of it that there can be no chance of mistaking it for anything else. Such descriptions are surprisingly rare.

Historical accounts of herpes are of little value unless they provide a good description of the disease, and it is obvious that much confusion existed both at the time of writing and in later attempts to interpret these manuscripts in the light of modern knowledge. Some idea of the confusion behind names and diseases may be gained from the fact that one of the words Arabic physicians used for herpes was '*nemlet*', which means 'the ant'. In France in the Middle Ages '*formica*' (Latin for 'ant'), '*formy*' and '*fourmi*' were used as names for both erysipelas and herpes.

If it is already obvious that the virus's first name is badly chosen, it is likely that the next few chapters will make it equally clear that its second name, 'simplex', is a poor choice too. 'Herpes complex' would have been much better.

In 1694 an English doctor, Richard Morton, wrote a very clear account of lip herpes and detailed its association with fevers, though unfortunately he did not choose to use the name 'herpes'. This is one of the best descriptions of the disease in European literature. It may seem strange that so few accurate accounts exist of such a common infection. This can probably be explained by the fact that such writings may simply have not survived or the accounts given are so obscure that they cannot be identified with certainty. This is most definitely true in the history of the genital variety of the disease. Naturally accounts of illnesses and diseases affecting this very important bit of our bodies abound, but once again obscurity of language and description make it impossible to identify with any certainty the first description of genital herpes.

Perhaps one of the earliest accounts was that of a French doctor, Jean Astruc, in 1736. It is of interest because he gave an excellent account of the disease as it affected the genital organs and actually classified the illness as a venereal disease. He also noted that it could affect homosexual men, again as a direct result of their sexual activities. Over a hundred years later another Frenchman appears to have been one of the earliest to draw attention to the fact that herpes could affect the neck of the womb. Many authors wrote about the illness in the middle and later years of the nineteenth century and most were aware of the fact that it appeared to be spread by sexual contact.

A number of doctors believed it to be very rare in women, though Unna, a famous German skin and venereal disease specialist, showed that, in Hamburg at least, it was a common infection of women. This belief may have been due to the fact that some infections of herpes in women may involve only the neck of the womb and as a result they would not be diagnosed unless an internal examination had been undertaken. Unna also noted that, in his clinic, genital herpes was quite frequently associated with other infections such as syphilis and gonorrhoea that were well known to spread from person to person as the result of sexual intercourse.

In the early to middle years of the twentieth century then, genital herpes was well recognized as a not uncommon but not very important infection of the genital region in both men and women. It caused two main problems from the physician's point of view: firstly, as it produced ulceration, it could cause difficulty in the diagnosis of the early stages of syphilis (genital ulcers are a common sign of early syphilis), and secondly, recurrences were common and little, seemingly, could be done to prevent them. With the discovery of penicillin and its widespread use in the late forties and fifties, however, syphilis became a much less feared disease. Patients infected with it were cured quickly and, even more importantly, became non-infectious more rapidly. As a result of these advances (and many other social changes) the illness has become a relatively uncommon one today. The other illness, apart from syphilis and herpes, which causes ulceration of the genital organs is the venereal disease called chancroid, or soft sore. This infection had started to decline in the early years of this century and, with the arrival of the antibiotic era it had become very rare in the United Kingdom, only some forty-two cases for example being reported in 1979 – and a proportion of these would have been acquired outside the United Kingdom. Thus, by the late fifties, herpes infection was the commonest cause of ulceration of the genitals in this country. Nevertheless, it was not very common, and in 1971, the first year in which cases attending clinics were recorded, they numbered 3,671.

The 'Sexual Revolution'

In the early sixties old authoritarian attitudes and views began to be questioned more and more, and this was to affect many aspects of behaviour. Foremost of these was sexuality, which, certainly amongst the younger members of the community, came to be viewed in a more relaxed manner. These attitudes coincided with the women's movement and advances in contraception such as the birth pill and the intra-uterine device. As a result the 'swinging sixties' and the 'permissive society' were born. The new contraceptive, the birth pill, conferred upon women an enormous freedom – for the first time in history they had a form of birth control which was entirely in their control and was virtually foolproof. Unfortunately, it did not interpose any barrier to disease or germs, as the old-fashioned sheath did very effectively.

This new freedom has fundamentally altered attitudes to many aspects of sexuality, the full consequences of which are not yet entirely clear. What seems certain is that this change in sexual attitudes, which has been given the rather emotive title of 'sexual revolution' by some, is unlikely to change back quite as much and as fast as history might teach us to expect. In other words, the pendulum is unlikely to swing back very far when the next change in our society's attitudes to sex and sexuality takes place, as it surely will.

Amongst the changes in sexual behaviour that took place was one that became an inevitability for many people, namely a more frequent change of partners. This does not necessarily imply sexual promiscuity, but if sex lives begin in the late teens or even earlier it is highly unlikely that partnerships formed at this early age will persist for life. Another feature has been a much greater willingness to experiment with differing forms of sexual expression and in particular with oro-genital sexual contact. This means, in simple terms, kissing the genitals. Thirty years ago this was considered almost to be a sexual perversion, while today it is a part of the sexual repertoire of many normal couples.

These two facts (increased frequency of partner changes and oro-genital sexuality) probably play an important part in the increase in genital herpes infections which began to be seen from the mid-seventies onwards. The influence of partner changing is obvious, while oro-genital sex would introduce another potential source of infection. Whereas previously only genital–genital contacts spread the illness, now oro-genital contacts would introduce an important new route of virus spread.

Another factor which has a part to play in the level of herpes infections is related to the age of first infection with the virus. When acquired in infancy or early childhood, many virus infections are usually relatively mild, though if postponed to adult life they can be quite severe. An example of this is infantile paralysis or poliomyelitis – in primitive countries most of the population is infected in early childhood and paralytic disease rarely results, whereas, if infection is postponed to adolescence or later, paralysis is a common sequel. The higher the level of sanitation, hygiene and general living standards are, the more likely it is that infection will not take place in early life as frequently as it used to. There is some evidence to suggest that this is what has happened with herpes infections. Fifty years ago most people met the illness as young children (usually of course as facial or lip herpes) and in most cases the illness caused was relatively mild and often mis-diagnosed – after all, young children often have temperatures and odd brief spells of sickness which are never accurately diagnosed. It is known that oral herpes infections do offer some protection against later infections with the genital strain – the genital version tending to be less severe in such circumstances. Tests of blood samples from young people today show that a far higher number possess no evidence of previous herpes infection than was the case thirty to forty years ago. In fact, a large percentage of young men and women today have no immunity to either strain of virus and consequently when they do become infected there is a much greater chance that the illness they develop will be more severe than it would have been had they contracted it as young children. That they failed to do this must be attributed to higher standards of hygiene, yet this has had the paradoxical result that many more of them are susceptible to the infection when they start sexual activity.

The increase in patient numbers with a disease like herpes is difficult, if not impossible, to arrive at accurately, and only a rough indication of trends can be obtained from what rather inadequate official figures there are available. These come from clinics for sexually transmitted disease throughout Britain. Patients who receive treatment from their own doctors or go to other hospital departments are not included. There is no doubt that many patients do seek advice from their family doctors over this matter, and official figures could probably easily be multiplied by at least ten. The increase in the figures attending the British clinics is however substantial, a total of 10,800 being recorded in 1980, which is an increase of 60 per cent over the figure obtained in the previous five years. The increase in the incidence of the disease is said to be world-wide and has attracted especial attention in the USA, where the situation has been said to be serious enough to justify the title of epidemic.

Herpes has been attracting attention from some doctors and the public since the mid-sixties. Hence some of the 'increase' might not be as real as it appears at first sight. It will however be instructive to look briefly at what it was about the disease that drew first the attention of the doctors, and later, inevitably, the public. Before doing this let us remember that, to most physicians, herpes, wherever its site, was not considered a very important or interesting disease. Students would be taught that it appeared and reappeared on the lips in some people who were ill from other causes, while the genital form was worthy of note only because of the possible confusion with syphilis. No special teaching about the disorder would have been given as would have been the case with such important illnesses as influenza or German measles.

The Virus and the Spectrum of Disease

In the early years of this century it was discovered that herpes was due to infection with a virus. To grow the virus turned out to be a difficult matter at first, as it had to be grown on the cornea – the clear window – of a rabbit's eye. This meant introducing suspected material on to the animal's eyeball and then observing the development of the typical signs of the disease. It was not a very practical or acceptable method of diagnosis and was soon superseded by using the developing or fertilized hen's egg as a means of culture. This was effective but rather expensive, and eventually the technique of cell culture which is used today was devised. Here living cells, usually from baby hamsters or fibroblasts from humans, are grown in tissue culture media and infected with the suspected material. If it contains herpes virus this grows rapidly and damages, eventually killing, the cells in a characteristic fashion. A positive result can be obtained in forty-eight hours or take four to six days. This technique enabled a much more careful and accurate study of herpes, and the various forms of illness it can cause in men, women and children, to be undertaken. It was soon evident that it was an occasional cause of meningitis and inflammation of the brain, but more important was its ability to infect newly born children, in whom it could cause serious and often fatal disease. Another discovery, or re-discovery, was the fact that recurrent attacks of herpes infections were able to develop in people who had high levels of antibody in their blood – substances which in most virus diseases prevented further attacks from taking place.

Then in the early 1960s two similar, though different, varieties or strains of herpes virus were discovered, type 1, causing oro-facial herpes, and type 2, being responsible for the majority of genital infections – a theory which had been proposed in 1922 by a German doctor, Dr Lipschutz. The viruses are often referred to as HSV1 and HSV2, the initials standing for herpes simplex virus.

Following this discovery came the association of herpes infection with cancer of the neck of the womb and more detailed knowledge of the various forms of disease the infection could produce when it attacked newly born children or the central nervous system in patients of any age. The ability of the virus to persist in the body for life was confirmed and its identity as the 'forever disease' was finally established.

The Media Move In

These facts, each worrying enough when considered singly, became in the eye of the media an intriguing mixture of disease effects rarely, if ever, rivalled by any other illness in recent times: it was spread or contracted by that most universal (and interesting!) of human activities, sexual intercourse; once caught it could not be cured; people so infected could infect, admittedly intermittently, any subsequent sexual partners; it may be a cause of cancer of the neck of the womb; in perhaps at least a half the total number of sufferers, recurrent attacks developed which in some at least seriously interfered with their sex lives. A final horror: it was capable of infecting newly born babies, and of those so infected many would die, while of those who recovered 50 per cent would be brain-damaged.

On top of all this, doctors in general appeared to be rather uninformed and uninterested in the problem. Victims complained that they would be told only that there was nothing they could do about it. As a result, the media moved in, firstly in the USA and eventually in Europe and the United Kingdom. A torrent of articles, radio and TV programmes appeared, reaching a climax in 1980–82. While each programme may have been designed to help and inform, the general result was for each to produce an ever-increasing number of anxious, worried people, some of whom were genuinely suffering from herpes, though others, equally concerned, did not have the disease at all. Those who had sustained attacks and had regarded them as the minor illnesses they really were often became distressed when they learned that, according to some, they were suffering from an incurable venereal disease. Fear of infecting sexual partners in such a situation led to difficulties in many relationships which could become too severe for couples to cope with, sometimes even leading to divorce. It was rumoured that some members of the 'permissive society' had begun to wish that they had never joined and that 'casual sex' was 'out' because it was too risky – a state of affairs which had not existed since the early years of the century, when the then reigning venereal diseases, syphilis and gonorrhoea, were virtually incurable and as a consequence were both common and powerfully inhibiting factors on sexual promiscuity. How accurate an account of the true state of affairs this is we shall examine in some detail in subsequent chapters of this book. By the late seventies and early eighties genital herpes could be truly said to have arrived as an important and troublesome problem.

CHAPTER 2

Viruses and the Herpes Virus

Viruses, which derive their name from the Latin word for 'slime' or 'poison', are the smallest known infective agents. They are capable of infecting nearly all other forms of life, from bacteria and plants to animals, and they are distinguished from other micro-organisms by a number of properties. The first of these is their incredibly small size. When they were first described they were known as 'filtrable viruses' or 'filter-passing agents', as they were able to pass through the pores of mechanical filters which were small enough to block or trap the passage of bacteria. The unit in which they are measured is the nanometre (abbreviated usually to 'nm'). A nanometre is a thousand millionth of a metre and an average bacteria is roughly 1,000 nanometres in diameter, while viruses range in size from 300 to as little as 10 nanometres. These sizes are impossible to visualize and it may help to think of the size of a human red blood cell, which is between 7 and 8 thousand nanometres in diameter. There is obviously plenty of room in cells for many virus particles.

Viruses are completely 'metabolically inert' outside a living cell. That is to say that they can exert none of the functions of living matter such as the reproduction of their own kind. Once they gain entry to a suitable living cell (and they are very choosy about which type of cell they will live in) the nucleus of the virus, or 'genome' as it is called, is capable of making use of some of the complex chemical equipment of the cell's own nucleus and directing it to prepare substances which are then assembled inside the cell to make identical copies of the virus. Naturally, this course of events is nearly always bad for the infected cell, which often dies, liberating new virus which then infects other cells.

Thus viruses really don't grow at all in the conventional sense of self-reproduction. They 'subvert' the cell's machinery to make copies of themselves and have no existence apart from the living cells they infect.

Another important feature of viruses is the genome, which contains nucleic acid in one of its two forms: ribonucleic acid (RNA) and desoxyribonucleic acid (DNA). Each variety of virus will possess only one of these two compounds. This nucleic acid is of enormous importance to all living things, as it acts as the carrier of genetic information, and in the virus it is what directs the host cells to produce the necessary materials to copy itself. One could say that viruses consist virtually entirely of genetic information wrapped up in a protective coat.

The actual structure of viruses is relatively simple – a core of nucleic acid surrounded by a protective coat of protein. Quite a number of viruses, in addition to the protective coat, also have an envelope, usually made of lipo-protein. The protein coat can be of a quite complex structure and the assembly of nucleic acid plus coat to form a mature virus particle may take many quite complex and beautiful forms. For instance the herpes virus is a roughly rounded particle, with its protein coat made up of a large number of hollow protein units. The whole is surrounded by a loose, 'baggy' envelope and measures about 100 nanometres – a medium-sized virus.

The appearance of the fully formed herpes virus particle can be easily seen by the use of the electron microscope, while a few of the larger viruses can be seen with a high-powered conventional instrument, though not much, if any, detail can be appreciated. The electron microscope is able to see smaller objects than the ordinary microscope, as it uses beams of electrons rather than visible rays of light and then amplifies them. Light cannot illuminate anything smaller than its own wave-length, and of course electrons are much smaller than these waves.

We mentioned earlier that viruses do not exist outside the body except as inert matter. In fact when they leave the cell the majority of viruses will soon decompose and 'die' if they do not rapidly find a new home, and herpes simplex virus is one of these. It is rapidly killed by soap and water, drying and most disinfectants.

The Other Herpes Viruses

The herpes group of viruses form a family which, like most families, shares a number of characteristics. There are over fifty of them and they can infect a whole range of different hosts, from domestic poultry, frogs and some monkeys to mice, rabbits, fungi and even oysters. Each virus tends to stick rigidly to its own host or hosts and not to infect any other.

Man is the host for five herpes viruses and it is very likely that most people reading this book have at least four, if not all five of them living happily in some part of their body. In the vast majority of cases, as far as we know, they are doing absolutely no harm.

Perhaps something should be said about these other guests, even though this book is mainly about herpes simplex viruses.

Varicella Zoster, the Chickenpox Virus

The name of the first will be well-known to all as the one that causes chickenpox – the varicella zoster virus. This is an oddly resourceful agent, as it tends to cause two apparently different illnesses at the beginning of, and towards the latter part of, life. Most of us are infected in infancy or childhood and then develop the common fever of chickenpox. During this illness, however, the virus makes its way to sensory ganglia in the nervous system, where it remains throughout life. As we get older, the level of immunity to the virus (which can be measured in the blood) decreases in many people. Why this happens we are not sure, but a common result is that if the virus travels back down a sensory nerve, usually to the skin, it may produce there the painful, locally grouped collection of blisters we know as shingles. Such lesions provide fresh virus, which, should it infect a person who has not had the disease, will cause chickenpox. Outbreaks of chickenpox occasionally develop amongst young nurses and doctors who have been looking after patients with shingles.

Epstein Barr Virus – the Glandular Fever Virus

Another of the viruses is called the Epstein Barr virus, after the British doctors who first described it while examining cells from the cancerous growth of the jaw region, usually in children, called Burkitt's lymphoma. Almost everyone becomes infected with this virus and in the majority it produces no, or at the most a few, very non-specific symptoms. In a few, particularly young adolescents, it causes the common 'glandular fever'. Most interestingly, in parts of Africa it appears to be the cause of Burkitt's lymphoma. The reason why this most serious event should occur in only a few of those infected is a mystery, and clearly an important mystery, for, if we understood why it happened, we could prevent some people from dying of the disease. One of the factors seems to be that in these people the body's defences are very inefficient, and it has been suggested that repeated attacks of malaria may be responsible to some extent for the weakening of the body's defence mechanisms. It is believed that this virus resides permanently in some of the body's white cells – probably the B lymphocytes (see Chapter 3).

Cytomegalovirus – Another Glandular Fever Virus

The next virus, cytomegalovirus (CMV, as it is almost universally known), causes cytomegalic inclusion disease in some infants and again is very widely distributed. It too can be spread by kissing and sexual intercourse and is now known to be a potential cause of damage to the developing foetus. It must be stressed, however, that once again most people infected with it will have no symptoms attributable to it and it does not appear to cause them any long-term damage. There is an important exception to this. In the last two years, serious illnesses, including a previously rare cancer called 'Kaposi's sarcoma', have been developing in patients in the USA. These have affected mostly very promiscuous male homosexuals, and the basic cause has not yet been identified. The seriousness of the situation may be gauged by the fact that 40 per cent of those infected have so far died. Two clear facts emerge from a careful study of these patients: (1) their immune defences are scarcely working at all, and (2) all show evidence of recent or active CMV infection. CMV infections are known to have the ability, shared incidentally by many viruses, to damage temporarily the efficiency of the body's defence mechanisms. Finally, some evidence suggests that CMV virus actually plays some part in initiating the growth of the cancerous cells which go to form Kaposi's sarcoma. That they are able to do this may be the result of the suppression of the immunological mechanism which would normally prevent such an event taking place.

CMV virus probably lives in a latent form in one of the series of lymphocytes or white cells and produces no signs whatsoever of its existence to the patient, though its presence can be detected by various laboratory tests.

Herpes Simplex Viruses 1 and 2

The other two viruses (if that is a correct description of the situation) are the two 'strains' of herpes simplex virus and, as they form the subject of the book, deserve special attention here.

Herpes simplex virus exists in two forms or strains – HSV1 and HSV2. In general HSV1 causes infections of the mouth, face and eye region while HSV2 strains infect the ano-genital region. The differences between the strains are quite considerable though not all strains will show this – in other words there is often a 'grey area' where a strain may possess some of the characteristics of the other variety.

In general, however, the genital strain seems to be a more 'toxic' or poisonous variety than the oral form. For example, when grown in culture on the developing hen's egg, it produces rather bigger plaques of growth than an oral strain and tends to kill the embryo. The viruses differ too in that they have different molecular weights and produce different results in the way they damage infected cells when grown in tissue culture.

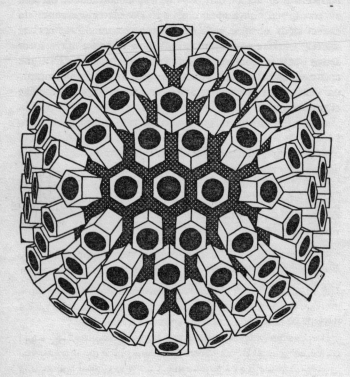

Fig. 1. *A diagram of the herpes virus capsid.*

Either virus is rapidly inactivated by drying and simple disinfectant measures.

When examined with the electron microscope, the virus is seen to have a relatively complex structure. The traditional scientific description of it gives some idea of this complexity but may not exactly produce a clear picture of the virus in the mind of the non-scientific reader! A diagram, however, makes, I think, the description comprehensible (Fig. 1). (The technical description describes the virus as consisting of 'a coiled central core of DNA surrounded by a coat composed of 150 hollow hexagonal and 17 pentagonal capsomers arranged in icosahedral symmetry' (a 'capsomer' is a protein unit which goes to make up the coat or 'capsid').) The mature particle is also surrounded by a loose 'baggy' envelope. In sections of tissue infected with HSV and examined with the electron microscope, the hollow capsomers, seen in cross-sections, produce a rather typical grid-like appearance.

The Diagnosis of HSV Infections in the Laboratory

HSV is extremely common in human populations and is almost certainly the commonest known virus infection. It is able to give rise to quite a wide range of different illnesses and has a particular, indeed almost unique, ability to cause recurrent infections.

Before we take a brief look at some of the patterns of herpetic disease in man, an equally brief look at the methods used for identifying viruses and virus diseases may prove helpful.

Electron Microscopy

With many of the larger and middle-sized viruses one can often identify viral particles in fluid, say from spots on the skin due to the virus, by using the electron microscope. This is certainly true of herpes, though it is in fact not often used for this purpose in hospital practice.

Immunofluorescent Staining

Immunofluorescent staining of material from suspected material is very accurate in skilled hands, though the reagents are both expensive and technically difficult to prepare. Basically, if there is any virus present in the preparation it will join up with a specific anti-herpes serum which is added to the slide holding the suspect material. This 'join-up' is then demonstrated by the material showing 'fluorescence' or 'glowing' where HSV is present when stained and examined under the microscope by ultra-violet light.

Tissue Culture

Tissue culture is the method most generally employed and the best choice in HSV infections. Some viruses, however, such as the hepatitis viruses, cannot yet be grown in this way.

In this technique certain cells from man or animals are grown, usually in a single layer, on the side of test tubes. The cells are nourished with an enriched and carefully balanced salt solution, kept at a temperature of 36.5°C and of course under sterile conditions. Growth is rapid, though after a few weeks some of the cells used will die off, while others obtained from embryo tissue can be used to inoculate fresh cultures and the process repeated many times. With tissues from certain cancers the process can be carried on virtually forever. Virus if present in these cells can be detected in a variety of ways, the commonest being the degeneration and, usually, death of those cells so infected. Other methods employ red cells, which stick to infected cells, as the virus has a tendency to agglutinate blood cells. Thus a positive result is produced when clumps of red cells are noted in the test system.

In the case of HSV infections, however, animal cells are often used as the tissue culture and a positive result can often be obtained in twenty-four to forty-eight hours, if growth is vigorous. More usually four to six days are required.

Blood Tests

All infections induce the body to produce substances in the blood called 'antibodies' to help to combat this state of affairs. Viruses are no exception and they usually cause large amounts to be produced, and, though it may seem rather odd, the antibodies often go on being made by the body for years, if not for life, long after the infection is over. So the mere presence of an antibody to a virus does not mean a patient's illness is due to that virus. The pathologist examines two specimens of blood, one taken near the beginning of the patient's disease and another some days later. If the amount of antibody in this second specimen is higher than in the first, it means that the particular virus whose antibody we are studying is responsible for this infection. Just finding antibody present indicates only that the patient has had that particular infection at some time (or of course he could just be starting his illness, in which case we could confirm our suspicions by finding a higher level in a second test a week or so later, which is just what is done to confirm some illnesses as being due to HSV infection).

Separate antibodies against HSV1 and HSV2 are produced and can be detected by specially sensitive tests, though in general these investigations are available only at hospitals with a special research interest in herpes. Tests in Britain showing antibodies to herpes in the blood nearly always refer to HSV1 infections and give no indication whether the patient has also had an HSV2 infection. The two varieties of tests for herpes antibodies are either the 'complement fixing antibody' test or the 'neutralizing antibody' test – the information they give varies slightly but from a practical point of view there is no difference.

Patterns of Infection Due to Herpes Simplex

Although we shall be dealing in some detail with the more important varieties later, we shall just briefly list the whole range of disease due to this enterprising virus. For the purpose of this list we shall not worry about which virus strain is responsible for which disease, as most can be due to either.

1. *Oro-facial herpes:* This produces the common, painful blisters on lips and nasal area which recur in many people.

2. *Herpetic keratitis:* Here the virus infects the cornea – the eye's 'clear window'. It is a very serious infection if not treated, and once again recurrence can be a problem.

3. *Genital herpes:* The sores or blisters produced affect mainly the genital and anal regions and are usually transferred from person to person by sexual contact. Recurrent attacks are a common and troublesome feature.

4. *Neonatal herpetic infection:* Herpes, when it infects newly born infants, tends to be a serious disease, as it often spreads to involve the nervous system and in addition infants have no significant immunity to the illness. Kaposi's varicelliform eruption is another form of generalized infection with the virus, but the brunt of the attack falls on the skin and it generally attacks infants with a tendency to hereditary eczema. It is rare.

5. *Herpetic encephalitis and meningitis:* Meningitis is a not uncommon complication of herpes infections, especially primary attacks. It may produce severe headache but rarely persists for more than a day or so. More serious is encephalitis, where the virus enters and infects the actual brain tissue (in meningitis only the meninges or cover of the brain is affected). This is much more commonly seen with oro-facial infections. No one knows why this occurs in many of the patients infected. It is an extremely serious, but fortunately extremely rare, disease.

6. *Herpes and patients who are immunosuppressed:* The immune system helps to protect us from infections. However, in two situations it is deliberately suppressed or poisoned by drugs: when an organ such as a kidney is transplanted, or in the treatment of certain cancers. In such patients, herpes infections – either primary or recurrent – can be most troublesome, as the disease has, as it were, an almost helpless enemy to attack.

7. *The association of herpes with cancer:* A number of other herpes viruses have an association with cancers in animals such as frogs, monkeys and poultry. Some evidence associates HSV with cancer of the neck of the womb (see Chapter 7).

We have now seen what a virus is, how they are grown in the

laboratory and how tests of an infected person's blood can be used to diagnose herpes. We have met briefly the large herpes virus family and been introduced to the five which infect us. We have had a somewhat closer look at herpes simplex and some of the illnesses it causes or is associated with. In the next chapter we shall examine the viruses' life-style in some detail as we see how the various herpetic illnesses develop and how the body tries to deal with them.

CHAPTER 3
Genital Herpes Infection: 1

In this chapter we shall try to follow what happens when the virus attacks the body and to give some idea of how the body defends itself. Most of the descriptions will concentrate on genital disease, but oral infections will be mentioned, as some knowledge of this is useful when it comes to understanding the complexities and ins and outs of infection in individual patients.

Infection Patterns

The first thing to understand about infection with herpes is a fact which is a rather difficult one for people who are not professional students of infectious disease such as microbiologists and doctors. This is that in the vast majority of infections with the virus, the infection actually produces no clinical illness at all – that is the person involved has no idea he has been attacked. In some, the illness produced is so mild that little attention is paid to it, or it may be misdiagnosed. We know that this is true because whenever an infection with the virus takes place, no matter how slight, antibody is produced and the body goes on making it for many years. Thus, by surveying samples of blood from a large number of people and then checking their medical histories, we can build up an accurate picture of how herpes behaves in a whole community.

Most of the studies of this nature relate to oral strains, or type 1 virus, largely because it has been known for longer and blood tests for it are easy to do. The figures show that at least 70 per cent of HSV1 infections are without symptoms – that is most people do not even know that they have been infected.

Such a mass of data has not yet been accumulated for HSV2. Most studies have been confined to particular groups of populations in very special circumstances and it is difficult therefore to use their findings and say that they apply universally. Nevertheless, when allowances are made for these factors, it has been estimated that at least 50 per cent of all HSV2 (genital strain) infections are also asymptomatic. Most of these infections, we believe, would have been acquired as a result of sexual intercourse, so such findings only appear in people who have started to take part in sexual activity. (As always, there are exceptions. In Nigeria for instance, small children have been shown to have antibody to the disease and it is suggested that the virus is able to move from body to body by means of infected objects (chairs, towels, etc.), the virus being kept alive by the warm, humid climate to permit some infections to take place without direct body/body contact.)

The remaining infections which take place with HSV do produce symptoms and we shall describe them shortly. Attacks differ widely in severity from person to person and we can only make some broad generalizations.

Primary Attacks

Primary attacks tend to be more severe in the adolescent or young adult than in the young child – as we have already mentioned, the same thing occurs with quite a number of other virus illnesses. Such attacks can be attended with generalized symptoms of illness, with a fairly high fever, aches, pains and a general sense of 'feeling sick', as in a flu attack. These attacks are often more troublesome in women, as they tend to produce more herpes sores and, because of the anatomy of the region, are often more painful as a result of the inevitable contact with urine.

There is another category of attacks which need not concern us very closely, but it is one of great interest to those studying the disease. This form of attack is called an *initial attack*. These patients give no history of a previous herpes attack and consult their doctor with what to them is certainly their first herpetic illness. Yet testing their blood shows antibody to the virus present in quantities that could only result from a previous infection, which in the individual concerned must have been a silent one. It is not clear exactly why or how these attacks develop, but it seems possible that re-infection may have taken place as a result of a very large dose of virus overcoming the relative degree of immunity that the patient possessed.

The primary attacks we have mentioned above as sometimes being severe are much outnumbered by attacks which are not at all severe. In most patients the cycle of soreness, itching, blistering, ulcers and healing takes only five to fourteen days to complete and is attended with no general symptoms at all.

Recurrent Attacks

Recurrent attacks are one of the most troublesome features of the illness, as they affect from 40–70 per cent of people and seem to be distinctly more frequent with HSV2 strains. The illness itself is less troublesome, lasting often only a few days, and the only general symptoms usually noted are neuralgic aches or mild pains in the area. Relatively mild as most of these attacks are, when sited on the genitals they can cause considerable pain, anxiety and worry to those affected. Such patients are of course infectious to others at this time by direct contact with the affected areas. (The problem of recurrence is dealt with in more detail later.)

The description given above applies equally to both oral and genital infection.

Method of Infection

The virus arrives at the site of infection generally as the direct result of body-to-body contacts. That is, one person has virus present, usually in a herpes sore and, as a result, live virus is then transferred to the other person. We should note here that the virus may come from mouth or lips and be transferred by oro-genital contact to the genitals. Equally, though fortunately not very often, virus may be present at either site in the total absence of any local lesions.

Before infection, however, the sufferer must be susceptible to the attack (that is have no immunity as a result of previous disease) and the virus must land on a site where it is able to get into suitable cells. The most suitable cells for the virus's purpose are those of the mucous membranes – that is those areas of 'wet skin' which line lips, mouth, gut and genital tract. Here they rapidly enter the cells by a process which we do not fully understand. The mucous membrane cells seem to have special areas on to which the virus can lock and then penetrate it. The envelope possessed by HSV also aids it in some way. To penetrate cells of the skin is a much harder task, and it is likely that the surface of these tough, protective cells has to be damaged to allow viral entry. Anyway, once inside the cell the virus makes its way to the cell's nucleus, which of course contains its own genetic machinery. This is promptly taken over by the virus, which employs its own nucleic acid to instruct the cell to start preparing materials which are eventually assembled into completed virus units. These units then move to the periphery of the cell, which incidentally makes a lot of virus material which never gets used in preparing new herpes virus. This activity usually leads to the cell dying and the release of mature particles of virus which acquire their envelope as they leave the dying cell to infect others. Each dying cell may release around 200 newly formed virus particles. (See Fig. 2.)

Most of the activity of the virus will be confined to cells in the area of this first contact, but a most interesting feature of herpes is that some virus almost immediately manages to get into the sheath of one of the myriad branches of the sensory nerves which are especially plentiful in such areas as lips or genitals (Fig. 3). These fine hair-like branches of the sensory nerves are the terminals of single nerve fibres which commence in a single sensory nerve cell. These sensory nerve cells are collected together in clusters which form small nodules or 'ganglia' and they are situated very closely

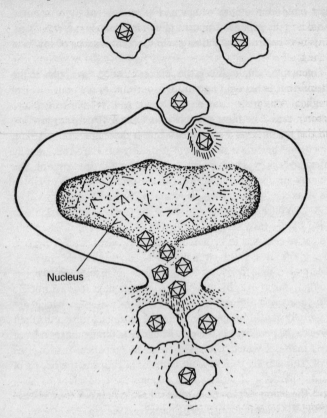

Fig. 2. *The invasion of a cell by herpes virus. The virus enter the cell, lose their outer coats, or envelopes, and then move to the nucleus. In the nucleus, viral proteins are produced and assembled into new virus particles, which then move out of the cell. As they leave they acquire envelopes. The cell dies.*

to the spinal cord, up and down the whole length of it (Fig. 4). One end of their single fibre is long and reaches to the skin or mucous membrane of, say, the lip or genitals; the other, a very short one, joins a fibre which runs from the ganglion into the spinal cord to form the first part of a chain which will eventually relay information about the state of affairs at that particular surface to the brain. The virus particles slowly travel up the nerve fibre (in the mouse the rate of movement has been estimated to be about ten millimetres in five hours), until they eventually arrive at the ganglion. There they appear to live for the rest of the infected person's life. We will return to look at this focus of herpes virus and the part it plays in re-infections later on.

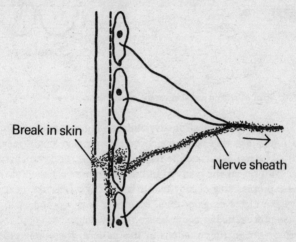

Fig. 3. *The passage of herpes virus through a break in the skin. Virus invades the underlying cells and enters the nerve sheath.*

At the site of infection most of the action is concentrated and the patient will begin both to feel and to see things happening there. The time from infection taking place to the first sign of the illness, the incubation period, varies a little but is around seven days. Many patients notice a localized 'tingling' or 'burning' sensation, which is soon associated with the appearance of a collection of small, red marks about the size of a match head. At about the same time the lymph glands in the groin on one or both sides may ache and swell. With mouth infections, the glands under the point of the chin or at the angle of the jaw may be similarly affected.

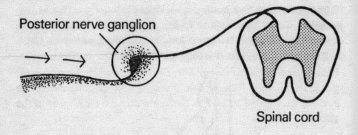

Posterior nerve ganglion

Spinal cord

Fig. 4. *Virus entering a ganglion via the nerve sheath.*

These spots become distinctly painful and rapidly swell into small red lumps like tiny boils, which quickly develop small, greyish-white blisters. The contents then turn yellow, and the covering breaks to reveal shallow, red ulcers which are very painful. This whole process may occupy two to seven days. Over the next few days the ulcers develop, then 'scab over', dry up and heal, the whole process taking about ten to twenty days.

There are many variations in this pattern, the whole process tending to be more severe, with more sores taking longer to heal, in those suffering primary attacks. In recurrences the sores may not ulcerate, there is rarely any fever and the whole episode may be over in a week.

In a few patients, and always amongst those with first or primary attacks, the virus may 'spill over' from the ganglia to inflame the nearby covering of the brain or spinal cord, causing a local meningitis usually marked by a severe headache and backache. Sometimes, in the case of genital infections, this may actually temporarily damage the nerves running from the sacral region of the spinal cord which are involved in the control of the bladder, bowels and erection of the penis. As a result the function of all these organs may be affected for some days, though recovery is nearly always rapid.

This sequence of events described above applies to all forms of infection with HSV1 or 2 with varying degrees of severity in different patients. The only difference that exists is that, in primary attacks at whatever site, the virus enters, for the first time, a sensory nerve and moves to the associated ganglion.

The ganglion involved in infections on the face are in the upper neck region, where several are fused together to form a large ganglion called the 'trigeminal' ganglion. In genital disease the ganglia are beside the cord in the lower sacral or 'tail' part of the spine.

The Body's Response

So that we can understand this more easily, a few words about how our bodies repel attack from micro-organisms will be necessary, as the situation is a complex one and not many readers will be familiar with it or some of the medical jargon that is unfortunately an essential tool for studying the problem.

The chief agents involved in the defence of the body against attack are mainly in the hands of the white blood cells, which have a number of highly specialized functions to perform. It is usual to divide the body's reply to infection (or its immune response) into two main arms, one of which can be crudely classified as, firstly, a series of chemicals which are present in the blood serum and which also includes such substances as antibodies which can be directly measured and are produced to order when the body is invaded. This is generally known as the humoral response, though the white cells are at the bottom of most of the activity as they manufacture the antibody. The second arm, or 'cellular immunity' as it is known, is undoubtedly the most important in dealing with herpes infections. The cells involved are lymphocytes of two varieties, plasma cells and macrophages, and each has a separate and very specialized function. Macrophages are large, white cells, though the name really means 'big eaters', which gives a clue to their function – they 'eat up' or digest what foreign matter they can find. Some wander or patrol in the blood stream and tissues, but in time of need they can be produced from the bone marrow in large numbers.

Lymphocytes – deceptively insignificant, small, round cells when seen under the microscope – are in fact very largely responsible for organizing and carrying out most of the attacks upon invaders of their territory. They are of two types and, as their function is so important and so different, we must examine them in a little detail. Their behaviour is one of the most fascinating aspects of human biology.

B lymphocytes are found mainly in the lymph glands scattered throughout the body, though some are always present in the blood stream. They are believed to develop and mature in various parts of the intestine and indeed owe their name of B lymphocytes to the fact that they were first discovered developing in a lymph sac or 'bursa' attached to the intestine of birds. When they 'recognize' an enemy they immediately begin to divide. Some are then transformed into an even more specialized cell – one with a slightly pear-shaped body and a large, darkly staining nucleus, indicating intense activity. This is called a plasma cell and it produces 'antibodies' specifically designed to deal only with the agent in question. Other lymphocytes appear to transfer news of the attack to the local lymph glands.

The antibodies that are produced stick to the invaders – in the case of virus infections, to the invaded cells themselves, and there they can have a variety of effects. One of these is to pave the way for the action of another chemical part of the defence system known as 'complement'.

The other collection of lymphoid cells, the T lymphocytes, so called because they mature in the thymus gland, are also very active cells indeed and are almost certainly of particular importance in dealing with herpes. At the first sign of infection they are directed to the site and on arrival they immediately start producing a series of different chemical substances (all with the usual difficult 'jargon' names, yet each having an important and practical function). The generic name for these substances is 'lymphokines'. One of these lymphokines converts the T cells into 'killer' cells by causing them to produce a toxin which kills cells invaded with virus. Others produced have the effect of speeding up the activities of the macrophages, making them work faster, while some other lymphokines, the macrophage inhibition factors, ensure that such activated cells remain and 'do their bit' at the site of the trouble and do not wander off. Yet another of these lymphokines has the effect of ensuring that any T cells 'passing by', as it were, are brought into the fight and are 'transformed' into active defenders.

The chemical 'complement' we mentioned earlier is in fact a complex system of nine separate compounds – all proteins which are present in the blood stream – and they work in conjunction with the system of antibodies produced by some of the B lymphocytes. These antibodies, as we saw, stick to, or coat, infected cells, and this union of infected cell plus antibody forms a 'lock' into which the 'key' of the first protein of the complement series fits exactly. Once this is achieved the others join in rapidly in strict order, until the final or ninth compound is attached. When this happens, the infected cells as well as the virus are destroyed, virtually instantly.

Another substance produced in the defence reaction is interferon, first described by a British doctor, Dr Alick Isaacs, in 1957. It is produced by infected cells and appears to help not the cells already infected by virus, but nearby cells which have not yet succumbed, enabling them in some way to resist attack. It is unique in that it is extremely effective, being active against all viruses, and has very little toxicity – that is, it does not damage normal cells in any way. Until recently a very scarce substance, new techniques of manufacture are producing sufficient quantities to allow it to be used as a practical agent in the treatment of viral disease.

The Defences in Action

The moment the cell is invaded by herpes virus, chemical messages are generated in and on the cell wall, which are immediately picked up by patrolling macrophages and B lymphocytes. The macrophages try to surround the cells, eventually breaking them down and later ingesting them. This activity attracts more of the same cells to help in the process and at the same time the infected and dying cells produce interferon, which does something to protect nearby but as yet uninfected cells.

The pace of the struggle accelerates, as some B lymphocytes will have acted as messengers by alerting T and B lymphocytes in the nearby lymph glands, which then head for the scene. Once on site some B lymphocytes will transform into the plasma cells, which then rapidly produce the appropriate antibody to coat the infected cells. This leads to the speedy activation of the complement chain and the early destruction of virus and cell. Further powerful help comes from the T cells, some of which, when differentiated into killer cells, join in the destruction of infected cells. Others produce lymphokines, which aid many aspects of the defensive action.

In the case of herpes, this battle is virtually always won by the body, though it may take many days. The time comes when cells infected are destroyed so quickly that the virus does not have time to reproduce, so that fewer and fewer cells become infected. Eventually no virus will remain, and this information will soon be appreciated by the white cells, which then begin to slow their assault with the lymphocytes returning to the lymph nodes, though the macrophages will be left to clear up the debris of the battle comprising dead cells of many varieties. At the same time, new body cells will be growing to replace those destroyed.

These changes, which we have described from the cellular viewpoint, can be related to the various clinical stages of an attack of herpes.

In the earliest stages the body's owner feels nothing. As more and more cells become infected the area begins to tingle, possibly to ache and soon the site of the battle between white cells and virus can be recognized as reddened spots, which, as the virus comes under increasing attack, causes these sores to fill with in-flammatory liquid to form the blister. The nearby lymph glands, warned to produce large numbers of extra white cells, swell up and also become a little tender. As the team of T and B cells, interferon complement, and antibody begin to make progress in their battle to get the upper hand, the blisters burst, leaving painful ulcers which rapidly crust over and heal where the defences have an easy win. In other patients, severe attacks may take weeks to heal up. New cells will then grow under the scabs, to replace the damaged skin or mucous membrane.

When this healing process is complete, a fundamental change has taken place in the body's attitude to herpes simplex virus. Its B and T lymphocytes now know it as an enemy, and some are programmed to respond instantly should they meet the virus any-where in their patrols around the body. Not only is this response rapid, but the amounts of antibody produced in the event of an attack are large. The patient has in fact gained some immunity to infection with herpes. Now in some infections with viruses, small-pox for example, this immunity is so strong that further attacks of the disease never occur. In herpes the degree of immunity seems to be extremely variable. Some will have no further troubles with the disease. Others will develop further attacks, though as the body is now 'primed' on how to respond to herpes attacks these are never as bad as the first.

CHAPTER 4
Genital Herpes Infection: 2

Throughout this complex sequence of events, we must not forget the virus, which has gained a safe refuge in the sensory ganglia. In many individuals, the next stage in the virus's assault is mounted from here, while in others it seems to use the ganglia as a base, causing no inconvenience to the host, but nevertheless emerging from time to time onto the surface, journeying there via the nerve fibres, presumably in the hope of being transferred to another host. Transfer to a new host is obviously an important aim for herpes, in addition to the basic 'viral drive' of replication.

It has been suggested by Sir MacFarlane Burnett, the eminent Australian virologist, that perhaps herpes evolved with man and is one of the earliest of his viral parasites or 'diseases'. Viruses producing short, sharp infections with subsequent immunity, such as measles and mumps, could not have existed in our early 'hunter gatherer' communities. There simply would not have been enough people for the viruses to 'move on' to to permit their survival. Herpes, however, comfortably ensconced in the ganglia, would move with man as he wandered about a largely unpopulated globe and, as we have seen, it is always on the look-out for a new host – such as children of the tribe or members of another group of humans who would be encountered from time to time. Such long experience has made it almost the perfect parasite of man.

We have already dealt with quite a few aspects of the problem as the patient sees it, but a little more detail is required.

Genital Herpes in the Male

The sores can affect any part of the penis and scrotum, though they are most often present on the glans or 'head' of the penis. Another common place is the fraenum – that little 'tie' of skin on the under-surface of the glans penis to which the foreskin is attached. In the uncircumcised male this part of the penis often suffers very minor damage during intercourse – so slight that it produces little in the way of symptoms. The important point is that the skin and mucous membrane have tiny tears which facilitate the entry of the virus. (The wart virus and the germ that causes the venereal disease syphilis also often enter the body at this point, so doctors are on the look-out for double infections.)

The sores, wherever they are, are painful when touched, though fortunately in the male they often avoid contact with urine owing to the anatomy of the area. When the glans of the penis is minutely inspected, especially shortly after sexual intercourse, small reddened areas and spots can often be seen. These are normal and are due to the local arrangement of blood vessels, which can easily be seen through the thin mucous membrane, especially when they are congested and swollen after sexual activity. Worried men often fear these are due to herpes or even syphilis, but they disappear in a few hours or so – remember, herpes spots are nearly always painful and persist for at least some days.

The glands in the groin are enlarged and a little tender, usually on one side only, though both sides can be affected. Aches and pains in bad primary attacks resemble those experienced with other febrile illnesses, as we have mentioned elsewhere. Sometimes a number of ulcers coalesce or run together to form a single, large ulcer which can make diagnosis a little difficult.

Herpes can infect the region around the anus, producing its painful sores in a ring round the area. Such an infection can cause extreme pain during attempts to open the bowels, and unless a careful examination is made there is a risk that the patient and the doctor will attribute the problem to 'piles'. The virus can also attack the inside of the lower bowel – the rectum – and produce a 'proctitis'. This usually causes a burning pain in the area and a discharge from the back passage. When the rectum is inspected after passing a small instrument into the rectum called a 'proctoscope', the typical blisters of herpes may be seen, but quite frequently the walls just appear reddened and inflamed – an appearance which is seen in many other infections. If herpes is suspected, the diagnosis is confirmed by growing the virus from a swab.

Genital Herpes Infection in Women

Exactly the same pattern of infection develops as in men, but there are important differences. One is that there are often more ulcers and they are very much more painful. This is due to the fact that the vulva has a larger area of very sensitive thin skin and mucous membrane, and, in addition, the passing of urine will wet many of them. This pain is then described by sufferers in such terms as 'as if acid was poured on me'. Indeed, so severe is the discomfort that when a woman describes the act of passing urine as 'agony', herpes is nearly always the cause, though acute cystitis or inflammation of the bladder may also occasionally be responsible. The fear of having to pass urine, with the resulting pain, may actually prevent some patients from being able to complete the act. Many, in an attempt to avoid having to pass urine, will stop drinking and eventually find they can only manage to perform in a hot bath, while others may develop the localized inflammation of the spinal cord and its coverings mentioned in Chapter 2. If this happens, in addition to the backaches and pains in legs and buttocks, many notice that the first thing to change with the act of passing water is that they have the normal feeling of wanting to empty the bladder but, try as they may, nothing very much happens. Eventually urine slowly trickles away and it may take minutes to complete an act normally finished in seconds. The picture will often be complicated with severe pain due to urine on open herpetic sores. In some, the paralysis is total and no urine can be passed voluntarily. Such patients usually need to be admitted to hospital for a 'catheter' or tube to be passed into the bladder to allow the urine to drain away. It may have to be kept there for several days or even longer, until the bladder recovers. If the opening of the urethra is covered with herpes lesions, the catheter may have to be inserted through the skin of the abdomen by a needle to prevent the risk of pushing virus into the bladder. This sounds a frightening procedure, but in fact it is extremely simple and painless, taking only a minute or two to perform.

Most attacks of herpes, even primary ones, are nothing like as severe as this. A patch of three or four sores developing on the skin of the outer lips of the vulva is much more usual, and here they will not be in contact with urine and, as a result, will cause little trouble to the patient except perhaps during intercourse.

The virus may also attack the neck of the womb. It is estimated that this actually happens in up to 70 per cent of patients, but most have no symptoms specifically related to the cervix. In some the cervix is covered in small blisters, which soon become smothered in a thick, greyish-white jelly secreted by the glands in the organ. The result is that the cervix looks a yellowish-white instead of its normal healthy pink colour. Such patients usually have a temperature and pain in the lower part of their abdomen in addition to any ordinary herpes symptoms they may have. Some herpes spots are often present outside but by no means always – the diagnosis cannot be made unless the cervix is examined.

Bad and moderately severe primary herpes attacks in women often temporarily 'paralyse' the local defence mechanisms. One of the commonest results of this is for a thrush attack to develop. Thrush lives in the genitals of many normal men and women without causing any problems. Once, however, it sees an opportunity to infect, it does so, adding itching and discharge to the misery already present as a result of the virus disease.

Herpes infections in women may be very localized and a favourite site is the anatomical equivalent of the male fraenum. The inner lips of the vulva run down and join at the lower part of the vagina in the mid-line. This, like the male fraenum, is a site of minor tissue damage during intercourse and consequently herpes often starts there. It may produce only two or three small ulcers which 'run together' to form a very painful 'split', which may cause such pain that intercourse is quite impossible. A similar state of affairs can arise from ordinary bacteria infecting small tears, so the help of the laboratory is usually required to sort out women who complain of repeated attacks of pain on intercourse at this site.

Oddly, infection of the walls of the vagina, though it does take place, is distinctly uncommon.

Recurrent Attacks

Recurrent attacks are a unique feature of HSV infections and between 40 and 70 per cent of people who have the disease will suffer from recurrences.

They can be frequent or very infrequent, though fortunately there is a distinct tendency for them to occur less often as time goes on, but there is no rule about this, the attacks persisting for many years in some people. About the only certainty concerning these episodes is the fact that they are always less severe than the original attack.

Apart from being extremely uncomfortable owing to their site, they can inhibit sexual activity because of the pain they cause or because of the fear of infecting a partner. As a result, various degrees of 'frigidity' and 'impotence' may develop. Others become very depressed at the regular appearance of the lesions, particularly if they happen to feel guilty about the circumstances in which they acquired, or believe they acquired, the illness in the first instance.

The exact reason why some people suffer recurrence and others don't is not clearly understood. To begin with there does appear to be a difference in the two strains, HSV 2 being more liable to recur than HSV 1. The factors which 'trigger off' attacks appear at first sight to be a very mixed bunch, with little, if anything, in common. They include stress, fever, local trauma, bright sunshine and menstruation, and these precipitating factors tend to be constant for individuals. Many people however experience recurrences and cannot attribute them to any specific factor.

As we do not know the reason, we must try to produce a theory to explain as many of the facts as we know them. The following theory is the one that appears to be the most satisfactory, but we must emphasize that it is only a theory.

One of the first problems we meet concerns the virus in the posterior nerve ganglia. It is known that virus, in the case of facial herpes for instance, often seems to make its way down the sensory nerves from the ganglia to the skin or mucous membrane at the site of the original infection. When it arrives there it does not always cause infection – indeed it is probably the exception for this to happen. Some idea of just how common 'shedding' of virus in the mouth is may be gained by the fact that mouth swabs, taken from healthy adults, will grow HSV1 in approximately 1–3 per cent of them. If those in whom no virus was grown are repeatedly examined in a similar fashion, in a month or so a quarter or more of them will have produced a positive swab.

Similar figures show that the same thing does happen in genital herpes, but again the data relating to these infections are not as extensive as in oral disease. What we have, however, suggests that it is rather less common and that there is a distinct tendency for virus to be shed less frequently and perhaps more importantly, in smaller amounts the further away in time from the original episode of infection one gets. There are unfortunately many exceptions to this broad statement.

Another mystery surrounds the state of the virus in the ganglia and what influences it there. Does it remain in a 'latent' or quiescent state until some, as yet undiscovered, stimulus switches it on to replicate and then travel back down the nerve fibres to the surface? Or does the virus continually reproduce in the ganglia, sending 'surplus' virus down the nerve more or less all the time in smaller or greater quantities? Or does the general level of antibody in the blood have some influence on the virus's behaviour? – it is normally considered to be insulated to a large extent from the effect of antibody in its home in the nervous system. Answers to these questions would help us to be a lot more definite about the recurrence problem.

The theory currently in favour which perhaps offers the best explanation of the phenomenon of recurrence in the light of our present knowledge is the 'skin trigger' theory, which postulates the arrival of virus at skin and mucosal surface from time to time and for reasons that we don't fully understand. When it arrives, it is suggested that either the amount of virus is too small to cause infection, or the body's local cellular defences (already primed and ready for such an invader by previous attacks) are able to cope. However, it is envisaged that some other factor is required to trigger off an actual attack in the skin or mucous membrane. The nature of this hypothetical skin trigger has not yet been elucidated, but on the basis of experiments it has been suggested that a chemical or group of chemicals called prostaglandins may be involved. The particular prostaglandin most likely to be involved is prostaglandin E2, which is produced in the skin when it is damaged (and this includes the damage resulting from the ultra-violet light of sunshine). It is also found in a high concentration in menstrual blood and is concerned in some way with the development of fever. Thus the theory is that if virus arrives at a site, say in the skin, in sufficient amount and perhaps the same area of skin has been damaged by sunburn or physical trauma to produce a focal concentration of prostaglandin, an attack of herpes may develop. If virus arrives at the site without prostaglandins being there too, no attack will ensue.

Even this ingenious theory doesn't explain why only some of us are affected.

There is, however, some evidence that minor defects in the cellular arm of the immune defence system may exist in patients who suffer from recurrent herpes attacks. These seem to affect some of the lymphokines produced and in particular the 'macrophage migration inhibition factor' seems to be both very slowly and poorly produced. This lymphokine is the one that prevents macrophages wandering away from the site of action. The killer cells produced do not seem to be as efficient as usual in their task of killing infected cells, and there is evidence that interferon production is not at the usual levels. These 'defects' appear to be specific for herpes – the defences work quite normally for other infections. Presumably they are fairly common in the population and are inherited. If this is the case, it would go some way towards solving the puzzle of herpetic recurrences, as these inherited, selective deficiencies of cellular immunity would often permit virus to grow and produce an attack of herpes. Often the trigger mechanism would be employed, but it would also be possible for attacks to start without it if, say, the virus 'dose' was large and the weakness of local immunity considerable.

Another theory is called the 'ganglion trigger' theory, which suggests that latent virus in the ganglia is, in some way, activated and spreads down nerve fibres to infect skin or mucous membrane cells, there producing a herpetic lesion. Unfortunately it doesn't explain how stimuli such as ultra-violet light are able to affect virus in the ganglia. Furthermore, as we have seen, the arrival of virus at the skin or mucous membrane does not always produce an attack by any means. Perhaps the biggest objection to this possible explanation is that in practice herpes lesions appear far too quickly after the precipitating events to allow the virus time to get from the ganglia to the surface, as the ganglion trigger theory demands.

When we do know everything about how and why herpes causes recurrent attacks, it is a safe bet to say that the process will turn out to be a fairly complex one involving many factors.

The Recurrence from the Patient's Viewpoint

Let us remember the following facts. Not everyone who gets herpes will have recurrences. Of those who do, these are never as bad as the first attack – in fact most recurrences produce little in the way of trouble and cause only an area of itchiness and minimal discomfort. In many, too, the recurrences are separated by long intervals, sometimes even as long as two or more years.

Some patients, however, do get very frequent recurrences which may occur with clockwork regularity. The site of the lesions is often crucial, especially in women – if blistering and ulceration occur and the affected area is so sited that urine may flow over it, of course the attacks will be painful. If in an area likely to be rubbed or pressed on during sexual intercourse, this activity will usually be so painful that the act is quite impossible. When one adds the very real fear of infecting a partner, it is easy to see how a person's whole attitude to sex can be altered. One such patient, a married woman of twenty-five years, who had been infected with genital herpes extra-maritally (an act of which she was deeply ashamed and had a tremendous feeling of guilt about), suffered from recurrences virtually every time she had intercourse with her husband. The attacks were locally painful and prevented further intercourse until healing took place, which in her case was after about ten days. She was then so upset, guilty and worried about the risk of infecting her husband that, as she expressed it, she was 'put off all ideas of sex for another two weeks'. Since she did not like intercourse during menstruation, she and her husband were able to make love only a few times a year, with little satisfaction to her. She confessed that in addition to all this she was 'petrified' that she would become pregnant and her baby would develop the illness. The load of unhappiness, frustration, guilt and misery felt by this poor girl is a typical result of some recurrent infections and is probably the worst disease mix the illness can inflict on us. Nevertheless such attacks are uncommon compared with the vast mass of silent and insignificant attacks made by the virus.

Self-Reinfection

Another odd thing about this odd disease is that a herpes sufferer who has recurrent attacks and hence some sort of immunity can actually infect himself at other sites on his own body with, as it were, his 'own' virus. If virus is taken from a lip or genital sore and rubbed into a scratch in the skin, say on the patient's chest, he will develop herpes there in spite of his immunity. It seems that the virus can overcome antibody in the blood and produce an attack. If the virus is inoculated into the same area from which it was collected, an extra attack rarely develops. This is probably because the cells in the general area of, say, the lip have acquired cellular immunity and it is this which is of paramount importance in resisting attacks with the virus.

What does this mean in practical terms for the herpes sufferer? Firstly the rule is that when 'open' sores are present, so is virus, which is capable of infecting susceptible partners. It is also capable on some occasions of causing self-infection elsewhere on the body surface. This normally requires the inoculation to be made through a damaged part of the skin. One exception is the 'cornea' in the eye. This 'clear window' is capable of being infected by contact, as are mucosal surfaces, so it is very important *always* to wash the hands after touching genital sores for any reason, which includes passing urine and applying ointment or cream to them for treatment. Far more importantly, if you are a contact-lens user and suffer from any form of herpes, never use saliva as a 'wetting agent' for them. Ideally, when genital sores are present, underpants should be worn in bed at night to cut down the slight risk of hand–genital/hand–eye contacts taking place during restless sleep.

If this sounds rather depressing, remember that most recurrences don't last for very long and that virus is present also for only a short time, usually only when the sore has ulcerated, and that this does not happen with each and every recurrent attack.

Recurrent attacks can present many difficult questions about such matters as the risk of infecting partners and dangers to others. One that not uncommonly raises particular difficulty concerns the couple who have been married, for, say ten years, during which they have been faithful to each other, one of whom then develops an attack of genital herpes. We shall asume it is the usual not too severe attack. It causes little alarm even when fairly frequent, but mild recurrences ensue until one 'learns' something about herpes! The worries about where it came from – 'was my partner unfaithful?' – and of transmission of the illness to this partner – 'will I infect him?' – can lead to enormous stresses developing in a marriage and to damage to the quality of their sex lives.

There are several explanations for the scenario, and all depend upon the fact that the other partner has had a herpes infection before. It may be one he or she knows about or one of the even commoner clinically silent ones. It may have been a genital or an oral infection, though, if the latter, the couple will obviously include oro-genital activity in their sexual repertoire. Equally the other partner may remember having had oral or genital herpes years ago – perhaps even before he or she married – and has had no recurrences since. In either of these circumstances, infection of a susceptible partner *could* take place if they had sexual relations at a time when the other 'silently' infected partner was shedding virus in sufficient quantity. Clearly this is very bad luck and very uncommon, but it does happen. One can reassure them that passing the infection back to the original donor of the virus, while theoretically possible, is very, very unlikely. The practical message is that normal sexual relations are in order, though obviously it is better to wait until any active sores present have healed.

Proof of a sort can often be offered to the couple of the previous existence of a herpes infection in the other, apparently unaffected, partner. His previous infection will nearly always show by the presence of antibody, so this can be tested for in the laboratory. As yet, in this country, the test is unlikely to be able to distinguish between type 1 and type 2 strains. Often, too, the pathology laboratory will need an explanation why only one sample of blood is sent for testing, for, as we explained earlier, they are used to testing two specimens, an 'acute' and a 'convalescent' serum, to show an increase in antibody and to allow a diagnosis of active, recent infection with herpes to be made. To them the knowledge that many people have had the illness in the past is a commonplace, and they sometimes wonder why a doctor should want to know such an obvious fact about a patient. Their slightly suspicious attitude is justified, as laboratories so often get asked to do unnecessary work by doctors who are not entirely clear in their own minds exactly what information they are seeking and why!

CHAPTER 5
The Prevention of Genital Herpes

Doctors are always being accused, with some justice, of being much more interested in curing diseases than preventing them. We shall therefore look at how herpes simplex infections may be prevented and how we can lessen the risks of passing them on to others, before considering the treatments available for this 'incurable' disease.

As we found in an earlier chapter, herpes simplex is spread by direct contact, which usually means body surface to body surface. In genital infections this implies genital–genital or oro-genital contact – in other words, sexual contacts and usually (but by no means always) sexual intercourse.

Some very recent work has also shown that herpes virus can survive for a number of hours on a lavatory seat and on cotton gauze (in one experiment it survived for seventy-two hours). This work does not alter the fact that the vast majority of infections of the genitals result from direct sexual contact. The long survival time of the virus in these experiments is nevertheless surprising.

We also learned that when sores are present the virus certainly is, so any sort of skin contact is 'out' in such a situation. Thus the sufferer from recurrent herpes should not have sexual relations when he has an attack – an obvious and indeed usually inevitable precaution, as the act of sex is so painful in such circumstances. However, many people with recurrent attacks get a warning when they are going to develop. This varies from person to person and may be an itch, a tingle or a burning in the genital area. These symptoms signal the imminent onset of an attack and appear to be directly due to the virus's reactivation and local attack. It is important to recognize them, as it is very likely that virus is present at such a time and the patient potentially infectious. This unfortunately rules out sexual activity until the sores have healed, and similar rules must apply to kissing anyone anywhere when lip sores are present. This is especially important with babies, and, should a mother with lip sores forget herself and kiss her infant, the baby's face should be immediately washed with soap and water.

People who suffer from recurrent genital herpes often worry whether or not they will infect a new sexual partner. As we know there is a risk of asymptomatic virus shedding and hence 'silent' infection, though this does not seem to be very common. When to inform the new partner is a difficult and delicate question, but he or she has to be told eventually. Some people, who are uninformed about the illness, could well break off the relationship when they are told that their partner had been infected, regarding the diagnosis as something akin to leprosy. However, when a relationship is established, the facts about the illness can be put in their proper context. This context must also take account of the fact that many sexually experienced people will have had herpes, even if they have no clear history of the illness (the estimated figure, you will remember, is around 50 per cent of all genital infections) and as a result are very unlikely to be reinfected. The rules about no sex when sores are present still apply, though.

Avoidance of genital herpes in the first place can be very largely guaranteed by having sexual intercourse with as few partners as possible. Clearly the more people one has sexual relations with, the more likely one is to meet someone who has herpes, which can then pass to you (possibly with other infections as well). As we have seen, oral sex increases this risk, as the mouth is another very important reservoir of herpes virus.

It is often asked whether a contraceptive sheath will prevent the virus from infecting the wearer. The answer is probably yes, but it is far from certain – the pores of a sheath are large enough to let virus particles pass through, so it is perhaps best to 'play safe'.

The combined effect of the advice given above may sound rather daunting and distinctly negative, but in fact the risks involved in sexual activity between two individuals as far as herpes is concerned are very small indeed provided no active herpes lesions are present. This seems to be the really important and most practical point in day-to-day prevention.

Whether oro-genital sexual contact should be stopped is a favourite question. The answer is 'yes, if one partner has mouth or lip sores'. Otherwise, if this is a part of a couple's love-making, it should continue and the extra risk, which is very small indeed, should be ignored. Anxieties about sexual practices of any sort are generally bad and can often be destructive of an otherwise happy sexual relationship. All acts carry some sort of risk – life is full of them – and it is neither practicable nor desirable to avoid them all. Avoidance of contact with herpes sores is both *desirable* and *practical* and all sufferers from recurrences should remember this.

The other odd feature we have mentioned about herpes simplex infections is their ability to be transferred to other parts of a sufferer's body, even if he already has a fair degree of immunity as assessed by blood antibody levels. Such auto- or self-inoculation is uncommon, but it does occur and the most dangerous place is the eye. It is surprising how frequently we brush our lips and rub our eyes with our hands or fingers. If these have recently been in contact with genital or lip sores, the virus can easily be transferred to the eye. Hence always wash the hands with soap and water (which will rapidly inactivate the virus) after touching herpes sores, wherever they are. If this is done the risk of auto-inoculation, already low, will virtually disappear.

Armed with this simple information every herpes sufferer can practise common-sense preventive measures, which do not interfere very much with life (though in some individuals, prolonged restrictions on sexual activity can cause havoc) but which do cut down very considerably the success of the virus's unremitting attempts to move on to another host.

For some individuals, the problem of recurrent herpes is a major issue. The fact that these individuals are relatively few in number in no way detracts from the importance of this problem.

Vaccination and Vaccines

Vaccination has been a great success in the prevention of a number of virus diseases such as poliomyelitis and yellow fever. In the case of smallpox, it has been the major influence in eradicating the disease. It seems that smallpox no longer exists, as new hosts for it, that is susceptible human beings, have all been rendered non-susceptible by means of vaccination, and the virus has died out. (This seems to me to be a little optimistic, but there is no doubt that the illness no longer occurs anywhere in the world. Whether it will make a come-back somewhere remains to be seen.)

What vaccines do is to employ virus which has been specially treated to ensure that it cannot cause the disease or other harm, and then introduce it to the body, usually by injection, in the hope that the body will respond as if infected with the disease. That is, a full-scale immunological response is produced, though without the clinical illness. As a result the body will then be very largely immune should it meet the virus itself, that is, if the individual is 'infected'. Some other techniques actually involve using specially modified live viruses which cannot cause significant clinical illness, yet do make the body respond as if they did – vaccines given by mouth in poliomyelitis are an example.

However, the behaviour of herpes simplex in producing immunity in those it infects naturally is not very encouraging. The immunity produced seems to vary very much from patient to patient and seems to be rather localized. For example we have seen that some patients with herpes, in spite of high levels of antibody, are still capable of auto-inoculating other areas of their body with the disease. We have interpreted this sort of reaction by saying that it is the cellular response that is the most vital element in resisting attacks by herpes. Thus the fact that effective immunity to the virus doesn't seem to occur very often in nature, if at all, is rather disquieting news. However, we do know that immunity does do something and can prevent infection if the infecting dose of virus is insufficiently large to overcome the defences mounted against it by the body's 'prepared' and 'warned' immune mechanisms.

Yet another problem of great concern in the preparation of any **vaccine** against a disease caused by a virus suspected of having the potential to cause cancer in some individuals is to make absolutely sure that the vaccine is free from such a risk. Added to this are the problems of reactions by the body to foreign substances introduced into the vaccine during its production – for example virus grown on fertile hens' eggs will, when harvested or collected for vaccine preparation, almost always contain some 'egg protein' to which some people may be sensitive, and thus reactions may develop after the vaccine is administered to these sensitive persons. Finally, the virus must be inactivated in some way – that is treated so that it is not capable of replication and actually causing the illness it is designed to prevent.

The History of Herpes Vaccine

The history of herpes vaccine production is not very encouraging. A series of vaccines have been produced in various parts of the world since the 1930s, but so far none has won approval by a substantial proportion of the medical profession, which suggests that they do not work very well.

These first vaccines were usually prepared fairly simply by the technique of formalin inactivation. The virus is killed by treatment with this chemical, yet, when suitably processed, it is safe to administer and still capable of inducing the body's immune system to react as if it were a natural attack by the virus and thus induce the changes resulting from such an event, that is, a degree of immunity.

These first attempts were not very successful in that patients still developed the disease and many of them failed to show any obvious pattern of increase in 'protective' antibody. Some twenty years later another such vaccine, which was used on children who had no antibody to herpes simplex virus, failed to induce the appearance of antibody. Even more importantly, the children – or a substantial proportion of them – eventually developed herpes infections. (Obviously these were all oral infections.)

Inactivated vaccines of similar formulae, usually against mouth strains of the virus, were prepared by some very reputable pharmaceutical companies, though controlled clinical trials failed to show any significant improvement resulting from vaccination and, as a result, most of these preparations are no longer produced.

One of the best-known preparations, which was used for many years in Germany, was a vaccine made especially for genital herpes, Lupidon G. This was made from a genital strain, propagated or grown on fertilized hens' eggs and the resultant virus killed by means of heat. It has been used in a number of clinical trials, several of which suggest it may have conferred some benefits, but the results were really inconclusive. The treatment with this vaccine was, in addition, rather drawn-out, injections being given over many months. There are obvious medical objections to repeatedly injecting foreign material into the body unless very positive results can be guaranteed, so it seems this vaccine will also fall into disuse.

More recently, experiments with a vaccine for herpes have been undertaken in Britain. Here, herpes virus type 2 was grown in tissue culture and then treated with a powerful detergent to remove the antigenic or immune stimulating proteins from the virus particle. (Many of these are situated in the envelope and coat of the virus.) The mixture is then spun at high speed to separate off the potentially dangerous viral remnants. These potentially dangerous substances are mainly viral genetic material. The vaccine is then treated with formalin as an added safeguard, as this destroys all genetic activity.

This vaccine has been tested and proved to have considerable efficacy in protecting susceptible mice against challenge with the virus and a little detail of what had to be done will illustrate the complexity of the experiments and point out some of the problems of 'moving facts in mice to facts in men'!

The experimental animals were adolescent mice, which were immunized with two injections of vaccine into the peritoneal cavity at two-weekly intervals. Some were given a control vaccine which contained no antigenic material – that is, it should not induce any immunity. Some time after vaccination, a piece of cotton wool, soaked in a live, standard suspension of virus, was left in each mouse's vagina for sixteen hours.

The infected or 'challenged' mice were then examined one, two, three and seven days afterwards. In each case a swab was taken from the vagina and cultured for herpes virus, while cells removed from the vagina by the swab were checked for evidence, and severity, of herpes infection changes. Under the microscope these changes are basically those which we have seen can sometimes be recognized in a 'Pap' smear as being the result of herpes infection.

The results showed that 'judged by observation (did the mouse survive or was it made ill by herpes?), cellular changes (an estimate of how severely the virus damaged local vaginal cells) and virus yields (how much, if any, herpes virus was grown from the swabs taken from the mouse after infective challenge) the vaccine afforded significant protection to experimental infection with herpes simplex virus type 2 in mice.'

The authors also found that if they inoculated the vaccinated mice with a larger viral dose, they were able to cause infection, presumably because the dose was large enough to overcome any vaccine-generated immunity – a general concept in herpes infections that we are now becoming very familiar with.

Interesting as these experiments are, they leave a lot of questions still to be answered, such as 'how long does the degree of immunity last?'; 'if the degree of immunity produced falls, how often will revaccination have to take place to maintain it?'; 'if given early, will it completely prevent the virus establishing itself in the sensory ganglia?' Finally, when we know the answer to these questions for mice, we have to answer them again for man and also to learn what, if any, untoward reactions have to be attributed to the vaccine. We have learned that almost every effective drug or medicine can produce such unwanted effects.

In short, it would seem that safe, practical, effective vaccination against herpes simplex infections in man is some way off – indeed it is not yet clear from the published evidence that it will ever be a practical procedure. However, experiments are being

carried out with similar vaccines in man and the results will be
studied with great interest by patients and researchers alike.*

* A recent preliminary report on the use of such a vaccine in men by Dr
Skinner and his colleagues at the University of Birmingham suggests that it
may have prevented primary genital herpes in a group of sixty adults
considered to be at risk from this infection. The subjects have been followed
up for a mean time of eighteen months, with a range from four to twenty-
four months of observation. In addition, all developed antibodies after
vaccination.

CHAPTER 6
The Treatment of Genital Herpes

There are so many aspects of the treatment of genital herpes that it could very easily form the subject of a book on its own. The experienced doctor knows that the existence of many different treatments for an illness usually means that none of them are of much value. The more that is written about treatments for an illness, the less effective these treatments are, would be a rather cynical, but not untruthful, way of summing the situation up. Until recent years, herpes infections and their management would have represented a classic example of this, although, as we shall see, things have changed and will probably change more than ever in the near future.

Problems

Before we look at treatment in some detail, there are two aspects of herpes infections which are in fact shared by quite a number of other disorders which make the assessing of any particular form of therapy very difficult.

Firstly – a universal principle which doctors sometimes forget – we are all individuals and we all differ very slightly in the ways we react. As we have seen, the herpes virus in man appears to be capable of almost infinite variation in the number of ways it will co-exist with us, producing a range of clinical illness from those severe enough to cause death, down a finely graded scale of severity to the vast mass of people who are unaware that they have been infected. When such variation is grafted on to the individual human, with all his specific problems and worries, it can easily be seen that to treat this illness in the fullest sense will almost always involve 'individualizing' the treatment. This of course is a part of the art of medicine, and doctors are constantly adjusting treatments to fit individuals. Simple, very obvious and rather mechanical examples would be to refrain from treating with penicillin an infection caused by a germ which was sensitive to that drug, if the patient gave a history of being allergic to it, and equally a heart transplant could be recommended for certain types of heart disease in a man of forty which would be quite inappropriate treatment for a man of sixty-five with a similar illness. The patient with a herpes problem has nearly always an individual problem which will concern many aspects of his personality, his social and sexual life, etc., as well as the actual disease caused by the herpes virus. If he could lose his physical disease – that is the troubles directly due to infection with the virus – he would usually lose most of the associated worries too.

Assessing Cures

Ill-health today is very expensive and so increasingly is its treatment. As a result doctors have become much more careful in making sure that expensive drugs really do work by ensuring that any trial undertaken is scientifically designed to produce results which really mean something. It is no good relying on the sort of hearsay that relates how someone's grandfather cured his arthritis with a herbal remedy bought in Wales!

The Placebo Effect

The word *'placebo'* means 'I will please' – and in a medical sense that is all a placebo is expected to do when it is given to a patient. Medically, a placebo is an inert substance which has no known or significant pharmacological effects, and it is sometimes administered to patients who insist on some form of treatment. The doctor does this, knowing that it can do no harm, and that it will 'please the patient', as he is getting what he wants. The odd thing, however, is that patients taking placebos often improve and improve very considerably. This placebo effect is extremely important, and the greater the faith the patient has in the doctor and/or the new medicine he is trying, the greater is this effect likely to be. For example, if one is testing a new drug, the patients receiving it may have great expectations that it will ameliorate or banish their symptoms. When this does come about for some of them, it is important to be sure how much is due to the medicine and how much to the 'placebo' effect. To avoid this, clinical trials, especially of drugs, are usually carefully designed today.

The placebo effect gives some idea of how the mind is capable of favourably influencing the course of an illness and, equally, having the reverse effect. Such knowledge can be of great value in coping with some of the stresses of herpes, particularly persistent or repeated recurrences.

The Design of Drug Trials

The most ineffective form of drug trial is that known as an 'open' trial, which is a very easy one to mount and conduct. The reasons for this simplicity are that no attempt is made to introduce a control group. All patients with the condition being treated are given the test drug, no attempts being made to ensure that they represent an accurate sample of those suffering from the condition. Nothing is done either to counter any particular bias the investigator might have – he may, for instance, choose only mildly affected patients or have a preference for treating patients of one sex. Most importantly, however, everyone in the trial will also be subject to the mysterious, but frequently potent, placebo effect. Such trials have little value from a scientific viewpoint, although, if everyone or no one is cured, some sort of point can be made.

The most effective form of trial is called a random, double-blind, placebo-controlled trial. The random choice of affected subjects ensures that a representative sample of sufferers from the illness will be chosen. The double-blind placebo-controlled design means that patients are divided into two groups, one of which receives the test drug and the other a harmless, inert, though physically identical, placebo. Neither patient nor doctor is aware of the identity of any patient's medicine until, when the trial is over, the code is broken and matched with the patients' records. Thus this scheme controls, or allows for, the placebo effect and will also do the same for any bias, conscious or unconscious, that the investigators may have. Results from such a trial, provided the numbers are great enough, can in general be relied upon. Obviously it would be risky to depend on the results of just one trial and usually a number of trials are mounted in different centres, often in different countries, in case factors such as race or climate play a part in the drug's effects.

It will be very evident that with such a tricky customer as the herpes simplex virus, any new compound purporting to cure herpes should be able to perform well in such a random, double-blind placebo-controlled trial. If not, any claims concerning its efficacy should be regarded with scepticism. Unfortunately, claims for herpes cures have not often been tested under such rigorous conditions.

There are several practical drawbacks, however, to such trials. They are expensive to run and very slow in operation, but in most cases the results they produce have to be accepted and eventually acted upon. As the results will eventually lead to the drug company selling or not selling its products to doctors, they will wish to ensure that their evidence is convincing, if for no other reason than to do otherwise would be bad for business in the long term.

Treatment

Treatment can be simply divided into *'symptomatic treatment'*, in which the physician tries to ameliorate the patient's symptoms – that is, for example, to relieve pain – and *'specific treatment'*, in which remedies are administered which destroy or remove the cause of the disease – in this case, herpes simplex virus.

This classification, however, does not take account of a long list of remedies which are certainly not specific and only help symptoms in a few patients. Most of these 'cures' come in and out of fashion, but the very length of the list is almost certainly a fair index of their ineffectiveness for most people. As herpes is a very individual problem, we will mention some of them briefly later as they may be of some help to some individuals. However, as specific treatment is likely to be the most effective and hence the most important, we will deal with this first.

Specific Anti-Viral Therapy

Everyone is familiar with the word antibiotic. The name is given to a group of substances which are capable of killing bacteria or of stopping them growing. The original substances were produced by other micro-organisms, especially fungi, but now many are synthesized or prepared in the laboratory.

These drugs work by interfering with the invading bacteria's metabolism – in short, they poison it, and to do this they must gain access to the bacterial cells. Normally there is little difficulty here, as most bacteria are easily accessible to drugs dissolved in the blood stream which penetrate and permeate every tissue in the body. There are problems – for instance penicillin does not cross from the blood into the brain tissues as well as we would like – but in general these problems are not serious and most bacteria are dealt with by antibiotics outside our bodies' cells.

Viruses of every type, however, live inside cells and must therefore be fought by drugs which actually penetrate the cell and kill them there. Ideally the drug should do no damage to the cell. If it did cause serious damage to many cells it would be too toxic for use, so it should also, if possible, be designed so that it works only in cells infected with virus, doing no harm to others which are not infected. At first sight it looks as if these properties would be difficult to achieve, and indeed such has been the case – viral antibiotics are a relatively new, though rapidly growing, branch of pharmacology. As we learn more and more of the intimate biochemistry of the cell, the more the ways in which we may be able to intervene in an attempt to interfere with the virus in its efforts to replicate become apparent.

Idoxuridene

In the early seventies a substance called idoxuridene was found to fulfil some of the criteria for an anti-viral compound where herpes was concerned. When it penetrated the cell it prevented the virus from reproducing. It was tried out in patients with herpetic keratitis, an inflammation of the cornea which can lead to severe impairment of vision and even blindness. It was applied to the cornea in a solution or ointment and was able to 'seep through' the thin, living cells of the cornea and enter the infected cells. It proved to be the first effective, topical anti-viral remedy and an effective cure for this dangerous form of herpetic infection. Unfortunately attempts to introduce it into the body for systemic use failed, as it damaged the normal cells' reproductive processes. When applied to herpes sores of the skin or genitals, it was of no use, as it did not penetrate the relatively thick layer of cells here. However, when dissolved in a liquid called dimethyl-sulphoxide, which has great powers of penetration, the drug did reach the affected cells and was shown to be a fairly effective local treatment for herpes. There were drawbacks to its use, especially in women, in that the liquid was difficult – if not impossible – to apply to all the sores, some of which were often sited internally. Also, some patients found the application painful. It worked much more effectively if treatment was begun within twenty-four hours of an attack, a target which was not often achieved in practice. Finally, the drug may rapidly lose its effectiveness once opened and/or improperly stored. It is also expensive. Worries have also been raised that repeated use may in some way damage DNA, possibly leading to the development of abnormal growth of cells, though there appears to be no evidence of this happening following its proper use in man.

It is available as 'Herpid', 5 per cent idoxuridene in dimethyl-sulphoxide, or 'Iduridin', with the same formulation. A 40 per cent concentration of idoxuridene in the same solvent is also marketed and has some effect on the lesions of herpes zoster or 'shingles'.

No preparation in dimethyl-sulphoxide should ever be used in the eyes. On the skin or mucous membranes it should not be used for more than four to five days at a time.

Since the introduction of idoxuridene, a series of chemical compounds have been synthesized and all owe their anti-viral activity to their ability to block viral growth in a variety of ways. These include such substances as 'cytarabine' and 'vidarabine'. Unfortunately these drugs also affect the metabolism of the patient's DNA, producing toxic effects when administered systemically sufficiently frequently to make their use a problem in a disease like herpes. They have been used with some success in the life-threatening situation of herpetic encephalitis, but they have no place in the treatment of oral or genital herpetic disease.

Acyclovir

However, it looks as though the star of the viral 'growth blockers' will be a similar drug to the ones mentioned above (chemically all are compounds known as 'nucleosides') which was first isolated in 1978 and given the name 'acyclovir'. The drug is a unique one in several ways, not the least being the very precise manner in which it does its work of inactivating the virus – almost as if it were specifically designed by nature for the task. It prevents the virus's replication but does not damage the host cell in any way. The drug becomes active only when it has undergone a chemical process known as phosphorylation, and this is carried out by means of an enzyme which is present virtually only in the virus itself – hardly any of the host cell's enzymes will phosphorylate the drug, so it remains inactive in uninfected cells. In addition, acyclovir also inhibits one of the main viral DNA enzymes responsible for viral replication while affecting the equivalent host cell enzymes to a much lesser extent.

Clinical trials have shown the drug to be remarkably effective in severe primary attacks of genital herpes when given by intravenous injection or by mouth. Pain and associated symptoms are relieved fairly quickly, while healing and virus-shedding times are greatly reduced. In one trial, virus in the control patients, for example, was often still present after three or more weeks, while patients receiving acyclovir shed virus for only five to seven days. In short, the disease was a lot less painful, it lasted a shorter time and patients were rendered non-infectious much more speedily. These results were all produced in impeccably designed and conducted trials and have been repeated in several centres in the United Kingdom, USA and Scandinavia.

Local treatment with acyclovir cream for acute first attacks was also effective as judged by relief of symptoms, healing and virus shedding, but as might be expected was not as effective as the internally administered drug.

The cream did not, however, seem to be very effective in treating recurrent attacks, possibly because of the relatively late start of treatment. Trials are now being conducted to see if the cream works more effectively if the sufferer has a supply of the cream, so that he can commence treatment as soon as he experiences the premonitory symptoms of an impending attack.

If the drug is given intravenously, the patient has to be admitted to hospital, and now that the oral preparation appears to be so effective it is unlikely that it will be used very much except in seriously ill patients. Given by mouth, the drug is taken in divided dosage over a period of five days and hardly any toxic effects have been reported so far. Some slight changes in kidney chemistry have been reported in a few patients. As the drug is known to be excreted by the kidney, care must be taken over dosage in patients with kidney disorders.

This, the first safe, orally administered, anti-viral drug to be effective in herpes, represents a great advance. However, all is not entirely straightforward. We know that, after treatment with the drug either orally or intravenously, recurrence develops in exactly the same way – that is the frequency and severity of recurrences developing are no different from patients who have not had the drug. Would long-term treatment, say for weeks or months, eradicate the virus from the ganglia? Would immediate treatment with the drug of all recurrences eventually either cut down their frequency or even stop them altogether? It is expected that such questions will soon be answered.

Difficulties are inevitable with any new drug and most of these seem to relate to unexpected toxic effects which may take some time to show or be recognized. So far no signs of any are present with acyclovir, though it is too early to say that there won't be any.

Resistance to the drug has already been reported in patients who have been treated with it and strains of the virus have even been found which appear to be naturally resistant. When the drug becomes available there is no doubt that the general situation concerning resistance will need to be very carefully monitored.

The drug also appears to be useful in at least one of the other human herpes virus infections, namely varicella zoster, though its possibilities have by no means been fully explored.

Finally, there is no doubt that, to begin with anyway, the drug is going to be expensive and this will clearly have some influence on prescribing for such conditions as recurrent infections.

Interferon

We have mentioned this substance (or more properly group of substances) which is produced by cells in the neighbourhood of any viral infection as well as by those actually infected, and how it appears to help cells to resist further viral invasion.

Interferon is a cell protein and is active only in the cells of the same animal in which it is produced – horse interferon would be unlikely to help humans fight infection! The great promise of interferon is that it is active against all viruses and is completely nontoxic. Apparently it causes a new protein to be produced in the cell and, while this has no effect on preventing the virus entering the cell, it seems to stop the virus from replicating. The inhibiting action on growth is confined to the virus, and the cell itself works entirely normally.

The drawback has been the very great difficulty in preparing the substance in a relatively pure form, making it an extremely expensive, indeed virtually impractical, medicine. These difficulties have now been overcome by new techniques of biological production and supplies will soon be plentiful.

The drug has been used against herpes as a local application in the form of a cream, with promising results. Properly controlled trials are being undertaken to see if this early promise is confirmed.

It would be narrow-minded to close this section on anti-viral antibiotics without pointing out the importance of these early arrivals for the treatment of viral infections in general. The previous rather defeatist attitude, that such drugs would be very unlikely ever to be developed, has gone and an air of some optimism now prevails. How interesting a compound must the new protein be which interferon causes to be produced! Could this substance, which appears to halt all viral replication without interfering with the cell, be the ultimate anti-viral agent?

Other Remedies or 'Also Rans'

This rather depressing survey of drugs has been made for two reasons – first to show how many avenues have been explored in the search for a cure, and second because it is certain that some readers will find that one of the remedies does seem to help them. As we have seen, there are several reasons for this, but the point at issue is that if they are helped by a drug (and it is not dangerous), they and their doctors should be happy. Doctors, however, will need very clear proof before suggesting it as a remedy for everyone. This list, by the way, is by no means exhaustive and is, as it were, a somewhat personal choice of both the most popular and the most notorious!

Influenza Virus Vaccine

Influenza has been a great problem to man, and indeed it still is. Vaccines have been in use for many years against flu and some of them are now reasonably effective. It was suggested that vaccination might act as a general non-specific stimulator of anti-viral mechanisms, perhaps especially interferon production, and that it might help in preventing recurrences of genital herpes. Some open trials suggested this might be the case, but the results of such trials, as we have seen, certainly in herpes, are meaningless. As the course of injections used far exceeded the recommended dosage of the vaccines, such treatment is *not* to be recommended. However, from time to time one sees patients suffering from long bouts of recurrent herpetic disease which appear to end abruptly following a single standard immunizing dose of flu vaccine. Though this is probably coincidence it may be worth trying, especially if there is a good reason for the flu vaccine anyway, such as a chesty condition or an impending epidemic.

Foods and Dietary Factors

There is no doubt that we are what we eat, and the truth of this statement becomes more evident as we very slowly learn more about the science of nutrition – perhaps one of the most neglected areas of study from a scientific point of view. Fortunately, there are signs that we are learning the lesson and many aspects of the whole vast subject are under active research.

Nevertheless, for the uninitiated it remains a minefield – diets are difficult to oversee or measure, and for a clinical trial with a dietary regime in herpes to be properly controlled is an exception. There is also a tendency to try to translate the results of dietary experiments on animals (which are easy to control) to man.

Obviously a diet adequate in calories, fats, carbohydrates, proteins and vitamins is essential for healthy life and especially so in the presence of any infection. This very mundane statement is really about the sum of our knowledge.

The following list of substances have all been suggested as being involved in some way (presumably by being deficient) in causing recurrent genital herpes. The reasons for the use of herbal remedies and yoghourt, for example, are even more obscure:

Vitamins: B complex, Vitamin C
Calcium
Zinc
Amino acids: arginine, lysine
Herbal remedies: seaweeds, herbal teas, etc.
Yoghourt

One look at such a list is hardly reassuring from a scientific point of view – indeed it suggests therapeutic desperation! However, something ought to be said about a few of them.

Vitamins

Vitamin C is a favourite medicine for a number of illnesses, including the common cold, probably because it is easy to obtain, relatively cheap and can be made into a very pleasant fizzy drink! However, it does have one particular property, namely that it cannot be made in the body in man and has to be taken in with the food. Shortage of the vitamin produces the illness known as scurvy, which was such a terrible problem for the Royal Navy in the eighteenth century, as the naval diet of salt meat and biscuits contained no vitamin C at all. Scurvy is almost certainly the only illness which this vitamin will cure. Nevertheless, and almost inevitably, it has been used as a remedy for recurrent herpes. There is a little experimental evidence to show that the immune responses are less effective in the presence of a severe deficiency of vitamin C, though this work was done on animals, not man. In short there is no rationale for its use or evidence of its efficacy in genital herpes. However, provided massive over-dosage is avoided, the vitamin is almost certainly harmless.

Zinc

This metal in minute amounts or 'traces' is one essential element of our diet. It forms a part of the complex chemistry of some important body enzymes and is present in cell membranes. It has also been observed to exert a slight but definite anti-viral effect on herpes viruses growing in cell cultures in the laboratory.

As a result zinc supplements of 50–100 milligrams daily were tried in recurrent herpes, and of course some people claimed they were helped. Again, there is no scientific evidence to support the use of zinc as a remedy for herpes. The supplements used are at least five times the daily requirements of the metal and toxicity is more than a theoretical possibility. A 'remedy' not to be recommended.

Amino Acids: Arginine and Lysine

These are two of the eight amino acids without which the body cannot function – the so-called 'essential' amino acids. Laboratory work has shown that in cell cultures an increase of lysine, with arginine levels kept steady, produced some inhibition of the growth of herpes virus. If, however, arginine levels were increased relative to those of lysine, the virus's growth was increased. A number of trials have been undertaken giving lysine by mouth and at the same time cutting down arginine-rich foods such as nuts. The properly controlled trials showed it to be ineffective and it is not recommended, nor are the diets which attempt to adjust the levels of the two amino acids. Such diets are unlikely to do any harm, but they are troublesome, like all diets, and they constantly remind the person eating the diet that he is 'ill' – after all that is why he is 'on' a diet and this enforced reminder turns up three or four times a day, at each mealtime.

The rest of the remedies mentioned above can be summed up by saying that there is as yet no scientific evidence that any of them confer significant benefit. If, however, a sufferer finds one of them that does help him, he should stay with it.

Local or Topically Applied Remedies

Again there is a large list of substances which have been applied to the sores of herpes in an attempt to achieve cure or relief of pain. Many were of course herbal remedies. Tea leaves applied as a plaster were well known, and even today the modern tea-bag, brewed and cooled, is still found to be a useful pain controller by some sufferers.

Ice

Ice applied to the sores of herpes is another folk-lore remedy. There is no doubt at all that ice does relieve the pain very considerably in some patients, but whether it has any effect in promoting healing is not known. It does not of course affect the frequency of recurrences. Applying ice to the genital area is not a particularly easy or practical manoeuvre, though it can be achieved with a small freezer bag repeatedly re-frozen in the ice compartment of the refrigerator. An enterprising female patient of mine found that a small pack of deep-frozen peas offered her considerable relief from the pain of a severe primary herpes of the vulva! As she put it later, 'One doesn't need a prescription for this and you can also eat the peas'!

Ether

This volatile, highly inflammable liquid, once used for anaesthesia, had a considerable vogue in the treatment of genital herpes in the late seventies. It was said to stop the virus's growth, relieve pain and speed healing. Ether is a very dangerous liquid for the home or laboratory, as its invisible fumes can spill over and, if ignited, track back to the bottle, causing a serious fire or even an explosion. Fortunately the controlled trial again showed that it did no good and it is no longer used.

Photoinactivation of Herpes Virus

This ingenious method first appeared in 1972. When applied to herpetic lesions, certain chemical dyes (known collectively as heterocyclic dyes), such as proflavine and neutral red, 'bind' in some way to any herpes virus present. If the area is then exposed for a short period to a fluorescent light, the virus, but not the cell, is inactivated. After the usual initial enthusiasm, worries about damage to the cell's genes surfaced, but once again careful trials showed the procedure to be ineffective, and it too has been abandoned.

The Treatment of Herpes Symptoms

Primary Attacks

The chief symptoms in a severe attack of herpes are feeling ill, local and general pains, and pain in passing urine. If the patient feels ill, he probably has a temperature and is better in bed. Local pain due to sores can often be helped by taking a painkiller by mouth, such as aspirin or paracetamol. This usually also helps the general feeling of malaise which so often accompanies any fever.

Pain on passing urine is usually seen most severely in women because the anatomy of the vulva makes it inevitable that some of the herpetic sores will be touched by urine during the act of passing water.

Some patients can be helped by applying an anaesthetic jelly such as Lidothesin to the inflamed area ten minutes or so before passing water. This, it should be stressed, does nothing to help the disease to heal – it merely allows the act of urination to be less painful to some patients.

In some women the flow of urine may be directed away from the sores if the act of passing urine is performed standing up over the lavatory while separating the inner lips or labia beforehand. Others find the act so painful that they can only manage to pass urine in a warm bath.

When healing starts, intense itching may precede or accompany this process. In women, as we have mentioned earlier, this is often due to a candidal or 'thrush' infection and will require the appropriate thrush remedy.

Serious difficulties with passing urine will often mean that a catheter may have to be used, in which case a day or two in hospital is probably the best way of dealing with the situation.

A few crystals of potassium permanganate (an amount about the size of a match head is all that is required) dissolved in a glass of hot water and stirred into the bath is an old-fashioned, though remarkably soothing, remedy. Care must be taken to dissolve the crystals, otherwise baths and bottoms may get stained brown.

There are some simple precautions that should be taken. The obvious ones of using one's own towel and washing flannel are most important. Cotton pants at night prevent or cut down the risk of any genital–hand, hand–face contacts during sleep. After using the bath, simple, thorough cleansing with a detergent will destroy any virus and the bath is safe for others to use.

There was at one time a considerable vogue for administering antibiotics or sulphonamides to patients with severe herpetic infections. The theory was that local bacteria had taken advantage of the virus's attack and joined in to cause a secondary infection. While this undoubtedly does happen, it seems to be fairly unusual, and the routine of adding antibiotics to the treatment is probably not justified, as all it does in many cases is to make the patient feel sick in addition to other problems.

Healing in severe primary attacks untreated with acyclovir may take three or four weeks, and of course no sexual activity should be contemplated until this healing process is complete.

Recurrent Attacks

All the therapies mentioned above may be employed in the symptomatic treatment of recurrent herpes. Because these attacks are less painful and shorter-lived than the primary onslaught, dealing with the symptoms is not quite as important.

The local application of an iodine preparation, such as povidone iodine paint or 'Betadine', helps some people. The paint keeps, is cheap and does not require a doctor's prescription. It should not be used if you are sensitive to iodine, of course.

Perhaps, as we have said, the correct management of these recurrences in the near future will be by either an anti-viral antibiotic or interferon, possibly applied locally or, in the case of the antibiotic, taken by mouth.

The Personal Factor

No remarks on the treatment of herpes infections of the genitals would be complete without referring to the tremendous influence our minds can have on our bodies and their diseases.

Stress can play an important part in determining the onset of a number of illnesses and recurrent herpes is certainly one of these. The problem is to define stress adequately. It is after all a part of everyday life and we are all subject to it. The sort of stresses that appear to be important vary with the individual but tend to be those which are severe and those which if not necessarily severe, are prolonged. Bereavement, the loss of a job or the break-up of a marriage are examples of stress which are both severe and prolonged. Chronic stress can result from a general dissatisfaction with one's role in life, one's work or perhaps especially one's sexual relationships.

There is some experimental evidence that stress can affect the immune system in an adverse way, while the placebo effect has shown us how the attitude of mind adopted by an individual can have very beneficial results as far as his illness goes.

It is common in clinical practice to see patients who are having a series of repeated attacks of genital herpes. In a few these can be almost continuous. Often it is found that they have coincided with, or been precipitated by, one of the unhappy, serious stress events mentioned above. Each attack reinforces the patient's feeling of hopelessness and depression. Attack succeeds attack, and there appears to be no way of interrupting them.

Many patients confess to a sense of depression and heightened anxiety when they realize that they are about to experience an attack. Sometimes the fear is a reasonably understandable one, as it means they are going to have to stop sexual activity for a while. Far more often the attack wakens all sorts of deeply felt anxieties, perhaps of guilt and of sexual inadequacies, or it may remind them of the result of their developing the disease and the unhappy circumstances it may have led to, such as the break-up of a relationship, or even a marriage. Equally, attacks may arrive at a time when a sexual relationship is coming under strain for a whole host of reasons. Women often secretly blame themselves for such a happening rather more frequently than men, and an attack of herpes in such circumstances can be the last straw for them.

We have already mentioned the mental turmoil that can occur when a sufferer from recurrent herpes finds a new partner (often after years of unhappiness following a divorce, for example), and begins again to contemplate the possibility of sexual relations. It is quite possible that anxieties about how to tell the partner, what the risks are, etc. may even generate some of the recurrences.

So what can individuals who suffer from repeated attacks of herpes do for themselves? (We assume they will have competent and caring medical advice.) Firstly, knowing and really understanding the common but very complex illness that they have. It is hoped that this book will do something to remove the worst of their fears about cancers, incurability and the dangers to babies. Secondly, this knowledge should give them some insight into the vital influence which stress and their own attitude of mind can have on the disease. A calm look at these factors and other current problems can often put a more cheerful complexion on what at first sight seems to be a fairly dismal situation. Thirdly, attention to general principles of health are never more important, though they may, for many reasons, be rather hard to achieve. These principles include of course a sensible diet, adequate sleep, exercise and recreation, and an avoidance of overeating, drinking and smoking. Fourthly, do see your doctor and tell him all about your problem – he is often in the best position to see if and when it has 'got you down' and that a significant element in it may now be a simply treatable depression. Fifthly, if you are the sort of person who can talk to others easily, try to contact one of the self-help groups formed specially for herpes sufferers. There you will be in touch with people who have your problem too and you can learn how they cope with it. Also such organizations keep up-to-date with all the latest advances in the field of herpes research and treatment. However, just talking about it to a sympathetic person who really understands how you feel can be of inestimable value. The truth of the saying that a trouble shared is a trouble halved is never truer than in this sort of situation.

Finally, try to adopt a positive attitude to your illness – it's there, you know about it, you have to accept it and live with it, as it lives with you. Such an attitude frequently brings about a complete change in the severity and even frequency of attacks. And, to look ahead: there *is* a strong tendency for the frequency of attacks to decline as time goes on, while the pharmacologists are undoubtedly going to present us with much more effective anti-viral remedies in the future.

CHAPTER 7

Herpes
and Cervical Cancer

The Cervix

The neck of the womb is a conical passage-way connecting the womb to the vagina. Its size varies considerably, but it is on average about 1½–2 inches in length and projects into the vagina, where it can usually be felt easily with the finger. Touching it produces a sensation very like that of touching the tip of your nose, and it is quite common for women feeling it for the first time to fear this 'lump' they have discovered is a growth.

The canal or passage is about 0.5 to 1 centimetre in diameter in a woman who has not borne children. During birth it has to stretch or dilate enormously to allow the baby's head to pass through. After birth the canal closes up, but rarely to the size it was formerly. It is lined with cells which produce mucous, a process which is at its height just after ovulation in the middle of the menstrual cycle.

Cancer of the organ develops chiefly in the area where the lining cells of the canal join the surface cells of that portion of the cervix which 'sticks out' into the vagina.

Like cancer in many areas it can be readily treated in the early stages of the disease but, if neglected, it can, situated deep in the pelvis as it is, spread widely to other parts of the body. Unfortunately, the early stages produce little in the way of symptoms, though at this stage it is 100 per cent curable. If, however, the cancer has grown to such a size as to be visible, the sad statistics are that roughly one woman in two will be dead within five years of diagnosis. Now, as everyone knows today, smears taken from the cervix can detect cancer before it is visible and can even detect 'pre-cancer' changes, so that nearly all cases of this cancer are in theory preventable, if women will have regular 'Pap' smears (after Papani-colau, who pioneered the technique) at the appropriate intervals. These intervals vary somewhat with age and the individual woman.

In spite of this, women are still developing and dying from the illness in the United Kingdom, and the annual death rate has changed little over recent years. Nevertheless, we have a low incidence in this country – 14 per 100,000 women each year compared with only 4 per 100,000 in Israel and, at the other end of the scale, a staggering 62.8 per 100,000 in Colombia.

A very worrying feature which has appeared in a number of Western countries has been the increase in recent years of cervical cancer in young women. The total numbers involved are small, but the trend is alarming. From 1968 to 1974 the mean annual number of women under thirty who died of cervical cancer was eighteen. For 1978–80 the figure had risen to thirty-one.

A similar and much greater increase has been reported in the numbers of 'positive' Pap smears in young women. The positive smears detect 'pre-cancer' changes, known technically as cervical intra-epithelial neoplasia, or CIN for short. Some of these do progress to cancer, but many will revert to normal if the patients are followed up. Much information is still needed about this group and they are being closely studied. It already seems clear that another common sexually transmitted virus, the genital wart virus, can be responsible for some of these changes.

To find out how this disease became connected with herpes infection is a long, complex and intriguing story to which there is as yet no end – it is still being 'written' by research workers in many different disciplines in many parts of the world. Perhaps the best way to tackle this problem is to approach it in stages in roughly the same order as these stages evolved.

The Association of Cervical Cancer with Sexual Activity

The first recorded observation on the association of cervical cancer with sexual activity was made by an Italian doctor, Rigoni Stern,

who in 1842 wrote a paper in which he noted that cervical cancer
was very rare in cloistered nuns and commoner in married than
unmarried women. He speculated that sexual activity was at the
bottom of these differences.

His findings on the rarity of the illness in nuns have been confirmed by many investigators, especially in recent years. Another
group with a low incidence of disease, reported by numerous ob-
servers, are Jewish women, and Israel has one of the lowest rates
of incidence of all countries, as we have seen.

After these initial discoveries, interest in the problem waned
somewhat until the 1950s, when a number of studies were undertaken to try to look at the role of sex, pregnancy and marriage in
the development of cervical cancer. What these studies basically
showed was that, when compared with controls, cervical cancer
patients were more likely to have had an early start to coital
activity, to have undertaken early or multiple marriages and also
to have had multiple sexual partners.

It was also shown that there was no simple association between
the disease and the number of pregnancies, nor with frequence of
intercourse if account was taken of the age at which coitus was
commenced.

Another obvious line was to look for evidence of cancer or pre-
cancer in women who had multiple sexual partners as a way of
earning a living – namely prostitutes. Not surprisingly both of
these conditions were found to be common in a group of such
women, and this finding has been confirmed by many investigators.

The Association with Sexually Transmitted Diseases

It was also predictable that there would be a connection between
cervical cancer and sexually transmitted diseases and this was first
shown for syphilis. Cervical cancer victims show a higher rate of
incidence of the disease than expected for women of their age and
class. Similar findings have been reported for the sexually transmitted disease trichomoniasis, while in 1974 Dr Valerie Beral

showed a really remarkable relationship between the incidence of syphilis and gonorrhoea and cervical cancer in the United Kingdom. She found this association held true for these diseases when the social class, the geographic distribution and even the occupations of the victims were considered.

One explanation for these associations could be that the disease could also be the cause of the cancer, but as the list of diseases lengthened it became more likely that behaviour was the common factor, an opinion supported by the fact that women of certain social classes and occupations tended to get both types of illness. Also, no observations were made linking syphilis, gonorrhoea or trichomonial infection in men with any particular cancer.

Nevertheless, the mass of evidence pointed increasingly to the fact that an agent, transmitted coitally, looked like being the most likely cause of many cases of this cancer.

Factors in the Male

If this transmittable agent did cause the cancer, there was a chance that it might affect the male, perhaps especially the genital organs, and several studies have shown that some men with penis cancer have wives with a higher rate of cervical cancer than would be expected statistically. This finding is not striking, however, and it does not seem to be a very powerful influence in men.

However, the sexual behaviour of the male does seem to be a very important factor in the disease's development, at least in some societies. In 1982 Dr Skegg and his colleagues from New Zealand published a study which set out to explain certain factors in the epidemiology of cervical cancer which can't be explained by female sexual behaviour.

They listed these factors as (1) the high incidence in many parts of South America, (2) the fact that, overall, the mortality of the illness has been declining generally in the West for about seventy years or more, long before the campaign for early detection by means of 'Pap' smears began, and (3) the often reported low incidence in Jewish women.

They believe that the male's sexual behaviour may explain most of these findings. They looked at sexual behaviour in different societies and suggested there were three main types. In what they termed a 'Type A Society', men and women are both discouraged from extra- and pre-marital relationships; in 'Type B Societies', men have many partners, but women are expected to have only one; while in a 'Type C Society', both men and women may be expected to have more than one partner during their lives. 'Type C' approximates to the state of affairs in many Western societies today, while 'Type B' is characteristic of many present day Latin-American countries and was almost certainly true of late Victorian Britain. Thus, in a 'Type B' society, many men will have intercourse with a fairly small group of women who will obviously concentrate any infections in the group, and, eventually, form a very important reservoir of sexually transmissible diseases.

Thus the high incidence in South America could well, in part, be accounted for by men visiting brothels and being infected with the cancer-inducing agent, which they then transfer to their wives.

The gradual overall decline in mortality in the West from cervical cancer is difficult to explain in terms of female sexual activity by postulating that over this seventy-year period women have become progressively more chaste, that is that they have had fewer and fewer sexual partners during this time! The authors suggest that a large part of the explanation for the decline could be that here men visit prostitutes less and less frequently compared with earlier times, so that fewer men acquire the sexually transmissible cancer agent and, as a result, fewer of their wives develop the cancer. Certainly such a change from a 'Type B' form of behaviour a hundred or more years ago to a 'Type C' is very evident today in the United Kingdom and many other European countries as well as the USA.

The low incidence in Jewish women was at one time attributed to the universal practice of circumcision of the males. In some way, the higher standard of penile hygiene so obtained was thought to lower the risk, probably by reducing the number of local non-specific infections, but this has not been confirmed.

Another significant fact contributing to the low Jewish risk has been the traditionally monogamous marriage, with extra-marital and pre-marital intercourse being perhaps less commonly accepted than in other societies. While this may well have been the case in the past, there is evidence that these older patterns of behaviour have been changing somewhat, while another factor may be that Jewish men do not seek the services of prostitutes very often and as a result will have a lower risk of all sexually transmitted infection.

Dr Skegg and his colleagues also drew attention to a little-known fact concerning carcinoma of the cervix sufferers originally mentioned in Dr Beral's work (which also highlights the 'male factor'), which is the higher incidence of the disease in the wives of men whose occupations involve much travel and frequent absences from home. The presumed implication is that, as a group, such men will be more likely to indulge in extra-marital sexual relationships as a direct result of their separation from their wives, with the result that there is, again, a greater risk of sexually transmitted infections and their consequences.

The other aspects of this study look at the risks for women who marry a man whose first wife has developed cervical cancer. We shall return to this later when we have considered some of the potential candidates for the role of 'cancer inducing agent'.

Cancer

Before we can deal with the possible association of cancer with viruses, let us remind ourselves exactly what a cancer is. We all know, that left alone, that is without treatment, a cancer is a mass of cells which goes on growing without pause. This causes it to spread, both locally by pushing other cells out of the way and by gaining entry to the blood stream and lymphatic channels, which carry it to other parts of the body where fresh growths of cells may be formed.

Why this happens in the first instance to an individual cell is not known, but a number of possible influences are. To begin with, a potentially cancerous cell is one which has in its nucleic acid incorrect genetic information, and if this cell reproduces, it will soon form a mass of similar cells. This incorrect genetic information, it is thought, could result from physical damage from one of many agencies such as radiation and certain chemicals. Equally, it seems very likely that every now and again, in the course of producing millions of new cells virtually almost daily for many years, the body will make an occasional mistake and produce a 'bad' cell, and that this is perhaps a much more frequent occurrence as we get older. Once these 'bad' or imperfect cells appear, the immune system recognizes them as such, begins its attempts to localize and destroy them, and probably succeeds in its task in most instances.

The other great problem with these bad cells is why so many of them go on growing in an unrestrained fashion. We do not yet understand this. Normal cells probably grow until influences from the nearby or neighbouring cells 'switch' them off in some way. This inter-cell information pathway, leading to the activation of the switch, appears to be absent in cancers, so that they continue to grow. The growth rate of the abnormal cells is unrestrained as a result of a failure of this switch mechanism. If, in addition, the immune defences fail, the cells will go on to produce a mass of cells – a malignant growth, or cancer.

As the mechanisms involved – the various possibilities of damage to the genetic material and the involvement of immune defences – are immensely complex, it seems likely that cancers are not going to have a single cause. In fact it is certain that there are many 'causes' of this disease. One that has been most studied is the possibility of virus infections damaging or subverting the genetic material of some of the body's cells and so setting in train the formation of a 'new growth', or cancer. This seemed likely to be a very productive approach, as, if a virus was responsible, a clear way of preventing the cancer could be seen – one could either try to avoid infection altogether, or produce a vaccine to prevent infection should the virus enter the body, or develop drugs which could kill the virus should it succeed in establishing itself.

Cancers and Viruses

The earliest cancers found to be caused by viruses were discovered many years ago in birds. The first of these was a form of leukaemia in fowls, described in 1908 by two Danish investigators. Then the 'Rous' sarcoma, perhaps the most studied of all these early virus cancers, was found, again in fowls. Since then the list has extended enormously and includes, to name just a few, breast cancers in mice, gut tumours in cows and leukaemias in cats. All seem to be caused by viruses with DNA in their genome (an exception is a group of 'retro' viruses, so called because of their ability to turn their RNA into DNA, which gives them tumour-inducing potential).

The changes leading to the cancerous state appear to start when the viral DNA joins with the DNA of the cells which the virus has invaded, and, as the cells' DNA is reproduced, the viral DNA is reproduced in exact parallel. Turning the normal cell into a cancer cell, or 'transforming' it, is closely associated with this phenomenon.

With such a pattern of events being so well documented in animals, it would have been surprising if the same pattern was not repeated in man, and this indeed proves to be the case, as a number of tumours are now known to be closely associated with viral infections. These include cancer of the liver with hepatitis B virus, the Epstein Barr virus with Burkitt's lymphoma and certain examples of cancer of the nasopharynx, and another 'possible' that we have already mentioned, Kaposi's sarcoma with cytomegalovirus disease. Recently, a rare form of human leukaemia, 'T' cell leukaemia, has been shown to be due to a virus infection.

It is noteworthy that two of the above-mentioned cancers are connected with herpes viruses – namely the Epstein Barr virus and the CMV virus. Other members of the herpes virus family are responsible for a mix of different tumours in animals – in frogs, fowls and monkeys – so that, all in all, this family of viruses has a fairly formidable reputation in its generic ability to produce tumours.

Shortly after 1967, when the two strains of herpes simplex virus were first discovered, it was also soon noted that the virus seemed to be found very frequently in the cervix and especially so in the pre-cancerous and cancerous cells of this organ. These findings were reported at about the same time as the associations between Burkitt's lymphoma, and a number of the animal cancers mentioned above, with various herpes virus infections were made. It was then a simple and logical step to look for evidence, particularly evidence of HSV2 infections as a potential cause of cervical cancer, as this could offer an explanation of the illness's association with promiscuity.

Direct cultures of the virus showed a high rate of positivity in cervical cancer when compared with controls, and a large number of investigations have shown a positive association with the possession of antibodies to HSV2 in the serum of cervical cancer victims, again when compared with controls. Not all the work has shown this, but the overwhelming impression is of a close association between the disease and evidence of infection with HSV2.

Perhaps some of the most convincing evidence for the role of herpes simplex virus has been the recent demonstration by some investigators that an HSV-specific RNA can be found in most cervical cancer and pre-cancer cells, but only rarely in normal cervical tissue. Other workers claim to have detected specific herpes simplex markers or 'antigens' in cervical cancers and pre-cancers, though very rarely were they present in controls.

Papilloma Viruses

Before leaving the virus question for a moment, there is one other virus or group of viruses that have been increasingly carefully studied in case they have a connection with cervical cancer. These are the human wart viruses or 'papilloma viruses'. They are capable of causing non-cancerous growths ('warts') of the skin, genitals, and larynx. Indeed one could truly say that is their way of life – producing tumours, albeit benign ones. Very, very rarely malignant change has been reported in warts at all these sites (and it should be stressed that here 'very, very rarely' means exactly what it says!).

In recent years it has been appreciated that the virus often infects the cervix, producing 'flat plaques', which in the past were probably ignored or dismissed as areas where a temporary and localized change in the cells was taking place. Wart virus can be identified in these flat lesions by a variety of techniques.

Warts present as visible tumours on the cervix are also common, but the appreciation of these flat areas as being due to the same cause is relatively new. These flat cervical lesions produce changes in the cells examined in a 'Pap' smear and these changes can be identified as being due to the wart virus. What is more important is that some of them are associated with additional cellular changes which in fact add up to minor degrees of 'pre-cancer' change or 'cervical intra-epithelial neoplasia'. It is not yet clear what the fate of these lesions is and a special study group of the Royal College of Obstetricians and Gynaecologists, set up to study the whole problem, was not able to come up with any definite answers. The two main possibilities, as far as the cervix is concerned, are that the wart virus changes may go on to induce cancer, or that the viruses' effects may be basically harmless, happening to cause cell changes which imitate very closely those early cell changes seen in 'pre-cancer'. It is known that some of the 'pre-cancer' changes seen in 'Pap' smears (and these changes are always mild ones) will often regress and clear up on their own, so it is possible that they are in fact due to wart virus infection.

It is obvious that a lot of work remains to be done before the part that wart viruses play, if any, in the development of cancer is clearly defined. Nevertheless, several authorities feel that, as things stand, they are as likely a candidate as herpes virus is.

One other possibility that has to be considered is that other, as yet unrecognized, infectious agents may be responsible. It is certain that other such agents, spread by sexual intercourse, do remain to be discovered (for example, we still do not know what causes at least one-third of the cases of the commonest of all sexually transmitted diseases, non-specific urethritis). This aspect of the problem has not yet been thoroughly explored. The lessons of Legionnaire's disease are still very fresh in the minds of most microbiologists.*

Other Possibilities

One other theory concerning the basic cause of this cancer which has a number of advocates suggests that it may possibly be sperm or, more properly, protein in the sperm. It is suggested that in the adolescent, when the cells of the cervix are differentiating and maturing, they are especially susceptible to attack. This attack is envisaged to be due to proteins present in the sperm heads of some particular males – classed as 'high-risk' males – and in some way this leads to the development of the disease. This theory has fallen out of fashion somewhat today, though it is by no means disproved.

Does Herpes Virus Cause Cervical Cancer?

In spite of all our inquiries we still can't give a definite answer to whether herpes virus causes cervical cancer. What we can say is that there is a very close association with the virus and the disease in many cases. There are also patients with the disease in whom no evidence of herpes infection can be found. This of course could have several explanations. One would be that the tests employed in looking for the virus are just not sensitive enough, and there could be a little truth in that. Another might be that the virus behaves very differently in different populations and in different parts of the world, but we really have no evidence of this. Another and more technological explanation could be that the virus does its dirty work and then runs away. In this 'hit and run' method

* An outbreak of illness which affected many American Legionnaires attending a conference in Philadelphia in 1976. A number of patients died. The disease was eventually found to be due to a previously unknown micro-organism now called 'Legionnaire's bacillus'.

the viral genome initiates, or switches on, the malignancy in the cell, but once this has happened the virus's presence is no longer required for the cancer's growth. It is difficult to prove and no evidence in support of it has been found in the case of cervical cancer.

One tremendously important fact is that many hundreds of thousands of women get genital herpes, but only a few develop cancer, so there must be other factors operating apart from the virus. We can only guess at these factors at the present time, but an obvious one would be the hereditary background of the individual and another the presence of other, perhaps repeated, genital infections. The age at infection and the state of the infected person's immune defences, as we have seen, could all be of crucial importance.

We mentioned earlier the work of Dr Skegg, implicating the male role in some cases of cervical cancer and referring to some most interesting work in progress in the USA, which shows that, if men who have had one wife who has developed cervical cancer remarry, their new wives are much more likely (about four times) to fall a victim to the illness than would be expected.

This could be explained in several ways. For example men may have a tendency to choose women with a similar background and habits for their wives. Another explanation could be that their sexual activities spread infection to both their wives. This infection could be a common one that could therefore be repeatedly caught and, as a consequence, have many opportunities to be transferred to other partners, in particular the wives, or it could be an infection which persists for many years, being intermittently infectious, which would ensure transfer to at least some sexual partners, especially wives. It has to be admitted that herpes simplex virus fits the bill very neatly – or of course the hypothetical, so far undiscovered, infectious agent!

What then is the risk of developing the disease for anyone who has contracted genital herpes? Almost certainly a very small one indeed, though certain life-styles might increase this risk considerably. Here one thinks of a promiscuous life-style, or perhaps a promiscuous partner, failure to have 'Pap' smears and so forth. An estimate in numerical terms has suggested that genital herpes increases the risk of cervical cancer by between six and eight times. When looking at these facts, it must be remembered how very small (relatively speaking) the number of cases per year in the United Kingdom really is. Six to eight times the risk sounds a lot, but when the risk itself is small the extra risk is proportionately small as well.

The other point to remember here is that this cancer happens to be one where preventative action can be taken by ensuring that regular cervical smears are done. With this simple precaution, nearly all the cancers can be picked up before they turn into true cancer – that is at the pre-cancer stage – and all, including the early cancers, are readily treatable.

The final message about this most disturbing potential effect of the virus on some of us is this. There is *no* such equation as 'Genital herpes infection = eventual cervical cancer'.

CHAPTER 8
Pregnancy and Herpes

Not so long ago pregnancy used to be a relatively straightforward sort of affair. The pregnancy started, progressed and resulted in a normal, healthy infant. Obstetricians were on hand to supervise the pregnancy should anything untoward develop which it did from time to time, but the end result was the same – the healthy infant. Today many mothers-to-be are worried when they become pregnant – 'Will my baby be normal?' is their major concern.

This is of course due to the much greater awareness today, following the thalidomide tragedies, of the risks to the developing foetus, especially during the early months of conception, and few mothers will nowadays accept medicines of any sort during their pregnancies without consultation and reassurance from their doctors.

With this knowledge has also come a much clearer idea of some of the risks of infections in the mother and the possible dangers to the foetus and newly born child. The front runner in the worry stakes over this aspect of the problem is undoubtedly herpes. All this is understandable. Pregnancy is a very special and unique event for the mother and her concern for her child can hardly be overestimated – indeed it is very difficult for the male to comprehend at all, though fathers-to-be quickly get some inkling of the depths of this feeling! Sometimes the feeling is clearly, indeed loudly, expressed, but quite often it goes underground and the woman worries silently about what might be going on in her body. It follows that many mothers are in need of calm, unhurried, accurate information about the particular problems which worry them most, and it is here, where herpes infections are concerned, that they can nearly always be given a 100 per cent reassurance that they and their baby will come to no harm as a result of this infection. However, it behoves us to remember the statistics about herpes in the newborn in order to get some idea of the anxiety such information may generate in someone who knows little else of the disease and its complexities.

The facts are roughly these. If a newborn baby is infected with herpes simplex virus of either strain, the resulting illness is usually severe, with a death rate of between 50 and 60 per cent. Furthermore, of the survivors, approximately a half suffer severe consequences, the most serious of which is probably brain damage. The figures relating to fatalities will almost certainly be improved when acyclovir (see Chapter 6) becomes generally available, though it is not clear whether it will have any effect in preventing brain damage. With this in mind, it is a little easier to understand a mother's distress if she is a herpes sufferer. If she is an informed herpes sufferer, she will lose most of her worries, and this chapter will set out to present all the information necessary to dispel these worries.

The Dangers of Herpes for the Newborn

The basic reason why herpes is a danger to the newborn is that such an infant's immunological defences are not fully developed or mature and do not work with anything like the speed and efficiency they do in the fully developed adult.

At birth, the child has a collection of antibodies passed to him from his mother's circulation. These have to serve him for the first three to six months of life, which is roughly the time it will take before his own system is able to manufacture them. Also, as we have seen, this sort of antibody, though it has some effect in preventing herpes, is not a very powerful one, and most of the effective defence against this virus is mounted by the body's cellular immune system.

Unfortunately this system is not yet very effective. The white cells – macrophages, T and B lymphocytes – function at a much slower rate than in the adult. Part of this is probably due to the fact that they are new to their tasks and have not yet met any of their main enemies. The whole process of being primed or warned about danger when they encounter it takes much more time – in great contrast to the rapid, almost violent reaction often seen in the adult.

Because of this weakness, the baby's defences are in many cases rapidly overwhelmed and the virus often enters the blood stream, which carries it to every part of the body, including the central nervous system. Such a massive generalized attack represents an impossible challenge for the body, and death usually ensues.

Then of course small babies, as a direct consequence of their smallness, are much more vulnerable to the general effects of any serious illness, regardless of its cause – toxins often overwhelm them, and oxygen supply is frequently critical, together with temperature regulation and fluid balance. All these 'weaknesses' are a general feature of many infant illnesses, and the skills of the paediatrician and nurses are well able to cope with all of them.

Herpes Simplex Infections in Infants

In general terms, herpes simplex infections in infants are rare. The figures we shall give may be somewhat of an underestimate, since very mild infections can be misdiagnosed, as – rather strangely – can some of the severe ones in which the typical blisters on the skin do not develop. Nevertheless, they are likely to give a fairly close estimate of the true picture.

In the United Kingdom, in the seven years between 1973 and 1980, only sixty-six cases were reported – less than ten a year. Much higher figures have been reported in the United States – amongst low socio-economic groups one estimate puts the incidence of neonatal infection with herpes as high as 1 in 7,500 deliveries, but this figure must be treated with some reserve and in no sense could be extrapolated to apply to the whole population.

Thus, the risk of a mother giving herpes to her baby in the United Kingdom seems to be a fairly small one.

We mentioned earlier that the numbers of infections with genital herpes is increasing and this could theoretically lead eventually to an increase in the number of neonatal infections, though there is little sign of this as yet.

Neonatal herpes can also be acquired from sources other than genital lesions and about a quarter of the reported cases are so infected. These sources can be maternal herpes elsewhere on the body, such as the lip, while nurses and others who have contact with the infant could be similarly infected and act as potential sources of disease. In one Australian hospital obstetric unit, for example, nearly one-third of the staff had one or more episodes of non-genital herpes per year, while 10 per cent of the staff without symptoms were found to be excreting the virus in the saliva. In spite of such findings, infections in hospitals are very uncommon. Staff who are suffering from active herpes infections are of course not allowed to care for infants.

There is also the risk that sick infants may infect staff, and in one American paediatric intensive care unit four of the nurses there developed primary herpes infections from such a source.

The Spread of Herpes Infection from Mother to Infant

Let us deal first of all with the very rare case in which the foetus itself is attacked while in the mother's womb.

It is known that a few infections, such as another herpes virus, cytomegalovirus, are on occasions capable of infecting the foetus by transplacental spread via the blood stream, but for this to happen the condition of viraemia, or virus in the blood stream, must have developed. This is very unusual with herpes simplex infections and when it does occur is almost always restricted to primary attacks, especially in those who are, for some reason, immunocompromised.

Even more unusual, it is believed that on occasions the virus may be able to make its way from the birth canal directly to the foetus, though this almost comes into the category of a real medical rarity.

From a practical point of view, perhaps the only slight worry for a mother is the development of a severe attack of primary herpes in the early months of pregnancy – any severe virus infection, such as influenza and of course German measles, can damage the foetus at this stage of development. The later development – later in pregnancy that is – of primary herpes we shall deal with shortly

In the great majority of examples of infant herpes, the child has been exposed to the infection from his mother during the process of birth. Over 99 per cent of babies whose mothers suffer from recurrent herpes are perfectly normal and protected from any risk of infection in her womb, though the moment the process of birth causes the membranes to rupture that protection is at an end, and any virus present represents a serious threat to the baby as it moves down the birth canal.

The most risky form of herpes from the baby's point of view is primary disease, for, as we have seen, virus is shed in larger amounts for a longer period – an average of two to three weeks. Also the cervix will almost certainly have virus present on it.

In contrast, recurrent herpetic attacks are of a much less dangerous nature, as the virus-shedding period is only a few days and it is estimated that the cervix is involved in only 15–20 per cent. Also the amount of virus shed is almost certainly smaller.

None of this gives much comfort to the pregnant individual, nor to her doctor, as infection is a real risk. Nevertheless, there is a rough relationship between the amount of immunity the baby has (from the mother) and the dose of virus required to overcome it and sometimes in recurrent disease it will work in the baby's favour. In primary attacks, this hardly ever happens, as the virus dose is so huge. Also, it is possible for a baby to be infected with herpes and develop only a mild illness, though one has to say he is probably a fairly lucky baby.

Recurrent attacks of herpes are in fact quite common during pregnancy – indeed some women find their recurrence rate to be higher than when they are not pregnant. There is no clear rule – some will have no attacks during a pregnancy.

We have mentioned primary and recurrent attacks and estimated the likely risks in each – a fairly simple task, as doctor and patient can see the signs of the disease. What is the situation when the difficult question of the risks of 'asymptomatic shedding' of virus are considered?

The fact of virus shedding in a silent or asymptomatic fashion is an incontrovertible aspect of herpes simplex infection in man, but quite a lot of controversy surrounds the details of the process, especially where genital shedding in women is concerned. For instance, the rates of such virus shedding in women who do not suffer from recurrent herpes range from 1 in a hundred to 1 in a thousand. Rates in pregnancy are unlikely to be very different from those found in 'random women', which are given in several studies at around 1 per cent. (This means that if one hundred women have viral swabs taken from the genital tract, approximately one of them will produce a positive herpes culture.)

Random shedding is unlikely to be a very important risk for neonatal herpes, as with these infections a source – usually maternal genital – can almost always be found. The development of neonatal herpes 'out of the blue', as it were, seems to be a very rare event indeed and this, remember, is out of a rare group of infections anyway. The reasons for this rarity are almost certainly the unlikelihood of shedding coinciding with the twelve or so vital hours of birth and the fact that the amount of virus lost is probably very small and that it is shed for a relatively short time, further cutting down the risk of infection developing. Also, if small amounts of virus are involved, as we have seen, even the baby's inadequate defences may well be able to deal with them.

Lessening the Role of Herpes Infection in the Newborn

Anyone who has had genital herpes should of course inform her obstetrician. He will be on the look-out for any lesions of herpes as term approaches, and of course the patient will report any signs or symptoms she considers to be suspicious indicators of an attack. In addition, many people now routinely carry out weekly viral culture tests from such women in the last three to four weeks of a pregnancy.

The whole object of the exercise is to prevent the baby coming into contact with any herpes virus and this usually means that if herpes lesions or positive viral cultures are present in the last two weeks of pregnancy, the baby is removed by Caesarean section to avoid risk of infection. In mothers at term who are found to have primary herpes, the same plan is followed, the only proviso being that the chances of successful prevention are diminished if the membranes have been broken.

It is known that viruses and bacteria can get through the protective amniotic sac or 'bag of water' once labour has begun, and Caesarean operations are planned to avoid this happening. The babies born in this manner will be entirely free from risk of herpes infection and as healthy as they would have been if natural birth had proceeded in the absence of any herpes scare.

It must be stressed that each patient's herpes problem is an individual one and has to be treated as such by her medical attendants, so that what is written above is only a generalization of what most commonly happens. Practising doctors are well aware of the fact that each patient's herpes presents a unique and separate set of problems, and perhaps nowhere is this more true than when pregnancy and birth are considered.

If a woman has had a Caesarean section for a birth because of herpes, it does not follow that all subsequent births must be by the same method. If, however, she has had several Caesarean operations, the muscle strength of the womb may be impaired by these surgical assaults, and the obstetrician may decide that the organ is just not strong enough to allow the baby to be delivered normally even if no herpes are present in a subsequent pregnancy. Once again, no simple rule-of-thumb answer can be given as to which form of birth is appropriate for women in these circumstances.

Finally, when a baby is born by whatever route and there is a possibility of herpes infection, it is usual for the paediatrician to check very carefully for any signs of the disease. The time the baby may be at risk or incubating the illness is up to twenty-one days, though the great majority will show signs of illness long before this.

Thus herpes infections, properly managed, are unlikely to lead to any serious damage for either mothers or their babies. Proper monitoring during pregnancy will allow those mothers at risk of infecting their babies to be selected for a Caesarean birth. This will prevent completely any infantile herpes.

The question of preventing herpes infections in small babies has been dealt with in some detail in Chapter 5.

CHAPTER 9
Special Problems

This chapter will deal with a mixed bag of difficulties connected with herpes, some of which have already been mentioned elsewhere. They include some details of infection in infancy, herpetic encephalitis, an account of the special problem of the disease in the immunosuppressed, and finally a brief account of the various forms of sexual dysfunction that herpes can on occasion contribute to or initiate.

Neonatal Herpes

We have seen why this disease is so frequently a very serious one for the newborn infant and have also seen how extremely uncommon a disease it is, certainly in the United Kingdom. It may produce a variety of disease pictures in the infant, and the form or pattern these take usually develops within a few days of birth, though occasionally it can be delayed for as long as twenty-one days.

Perhaps the most important fact to be noted is that quite a few infants with the illness do not develop skin lesions typical of herpes and therefore doctors will be alert to the possibility that any serious illness in a newborn baby of a mother with a history of recurrent herpes could be due to the virus. Early diagnosis before the child is very ill is obviously important.

In the disseminated form of the disease the clinical picture is that of a very serious, overwhelming infection closely resembling that produced by a bacterial infection which gains entry to the blood stream to produce a septicaemia. This is exactly what happens with the virus, and many organs in the body are infected as a result. Of these the liver and spleen are nearly always involved and their enlargement or swelling can easily be felt. The prognosis in these infants is generally very poor.

In the next type the infant is not acutely ill at first but soon develops a low-grade persistent fever and lethargy, and eventually fits may appear. The general tone of the child's muscles is poor and they are often described as being 'floppy'. Their livers and spleen are not enlarged as a rule and again many do not have skin lesions.

In the remaining type the infant's illness usually presents the typical sores of herpes. They may be one or two or very many, and they may be accompanied by signs of systemic infection. The worry is always that other vital organs may also be infected and early diagnosis and treatment is essential.

The outlook for many of these babies has probably been greatly improved with the introduction of acyclovir, though as yet no trials attest to its effectiveness in infants. The worries over whether the drug will prevent brain damage once encephalitis or infection of the brain has been established remain to be resolved.

Alarming as these aspects of the infections are, we must not forget how very rare (or how very important) they are. All babies born in this country have access to the care and help of skilled paediatricians, so that mothers may worry less when they realize that their infants are in very good hands.

Herpetic Encephalitis

We referred to this as one of the medical horrors, and it must be stressed that it is an extremely uncommon condition. Most infections seem to be due to type 1 herpes simplex virus, and cases due to type 2 are uncommon. What makes it a horror is the extreme seriousness of the condition and the fact that we do not clearly understand why it occurs.

Cases of the disease in Britain are rare – it has been estimated that up to sixty cases may occur yearly in this country and that nearly half of them will die. The fate of the survivors may be grim indeed, as severe residual brain damage is so common.

Although the factors underlying the development of this, the severest complication of herpes, are not understood, it seems clear that most cases probably originate from oro-facial infections, where the virus resides in the especially large sensory ganglion called the trigeminal ganglion. It is from here that it probably makes its way into the brain. Whether this is an accident – the virus, as it were, taking a wrong direction – or whether it is due to a sudden burst of viral replication in the ganglion and it 'overflows' into the nearby central nervous system and the brain is not known.

Once there, the severity of the infection of course varies markedly from patient to patient. The same pattern of defence that we saw in mouth or genital herpes is mounted by the body, with the usual responses by the immune defences leading to local inflammatory changes and the death of many cells. Unfortunately, the site of this particular battleground is a very different one from the skin. The brain is tightly enclosed in a rigid box, the skull, which gives it little, if any, room to expand, and, as a result of the herpes infection, there is a great deal of inflammatory swelling of the brain and its supporting tissues. This leads to high intra-cranial pressures which have all sorts of unwanted effects.

The other big difference is that brain cells are unique in the body in that they are so specialized that they have lost the power of reproduction and when they are killed they cannot replace themselves, unlike the skin or mucous membranes, where any gaps resulting from an attack of herpes are soon filled and complete healing results.

The common result is that, as the viral infection progresses, the intra-cranial pressure rises and these two influences lead to the gradual and usually disastrous death of many irreplaceable brain cells. This sort of sporadic herpes encephalitis can attack at any age, but is perhaps commoner in adults.

The disease also presents another major problem, that is of diagnosis. As we shall see the illness frequently starts with relatively minor symptoms and then slowly progresses, and it is often some time before it is appreciated that the patient is in fact seriously ill. The original physician – usually the general practitioner – is probably as likely to meet a case of herpetic encephalitis as he is to win a major pools prize, so it is not going to be one of the first diagnoses considered when the illness first shows its hand. Indeed, these first symptoms are usually non-specific, such as temperature, a feeling of illness or malaise and a headache, which is usually a bad one. These symptoms persist and are soon joined by more sinister ones such as changes in the patient's personality, by difficulties in speech and often by a sort of general confusion and lethargy – the patient is not quite sure where he is and is 'disorientated'. Accompanying this is a general weakness and frequently fits. Finally coma may ensue and the patient may never recover.

The realization that the patient is seriously ill leads to admission to hospital, but even there precise diagnosis is not easy. The virus can be cultured only rarely from a sample of the cerebrospinal fluid, which usually shows abnormalities, though they are not specific for herpes. Brain X-rays, angiograms and brain scans can provide information leading to the diagnosis being considered, as can the electro-encephalogram, which is always abnormal. The only sure way of diagnosis is to perform a brain biopsy and remove a small portion of brain tissue, usually from the temporal lobe. The cellular picture presented under the microscope is so typical that experts can make a confident diagnosis within thirty minutes or so of the biopsy being performed. In most cases the virus can also be cultured from the sample.

The brain biopsy consists of drilling a small hole in the side of the skull bone and passing a needle into the brain to remove a small fragment of tissue – not a dangerous operation, but one that is undertaken only when such a serious illness as herpetic encephalitis is being considered. There are many causes of encephalitis and, with the advent of acyclovir, we have a drug which may be of great value, so speed in reaching a precise diagnosis, and hence starting treatment early, is essential, as precious brain cells are being destroyed all the time.

So let us leave this, the worst that the virus can do to us, on a slightly optimistic note by remembering that it is a very very rare event indeed, and even here early treatment will sometimes be effective.

Herpes in the Immunosuppressed

Modern medical science, which has made so many advances in so many directions, has also introduced, as a direct result of these advances, some new problems which we did not have to cope with before. The serious infections herpes can produce in patients who are 'immunosuppressed' were hardly ever seen until the advent of the surgical technique of organ transplantation.

When an organ, such as a kidney, is placed in a new body and, with impeccable surgical techniques, provided with all the support and blood supply it needs, all is at first apparently well. But from the moment that kidney is in contact with the recipient's blood supply, the organ is immediately recognized as 'foreign' by the body immune defences and an all-out attack is rapidly mounted by all branches of these defences, just as we have seen how they attack the herpes-virus-infected cells. Indeed, it is not too fanciful to say that the kidney is treated just as if it were a very large germ or virus particle and every effort is made to kick it out!

These efforts can be remarkably powerful, so powerful in fact that organs can be so badly damaged that they have to be removed after a few days. This reaction by the body proved to be the biggest difficulty the transplant surgeons had to face, and they have still by no means completely disposed of it. The problem has been conquered sufficiently to make the operations a practical proposition and the story is one that is probably familiar to most readers. Firstly great care has to be taken to choose an organ from a donor who had a similar tissue type to the recipient. (Just as there are blood groups it has been found that tissues can be grouped in a series of types, though these are more complex than blood groups.) Even a perfect match will not stop the immune system spotting little differences and acting accordingly by treating the organ as a 'foreigner', though it may take some time to do this.

Thus more powerful measures have to be taken, which means trying to curb the body's immune defences. This has to be done by drugs which suppress or poison its activities. A whole host of such drugs can slow or stop lymphocytes working properly, and delay or stop the production of antibodies, macrophages and other white cells.

When such a paralysis of the immune system has been achieved, the new transplanted organ will be left alone. Unfortunately so will invading micro-organisms, so such patients will be under a constant threat from infections of all sorts.

A similar situation, that is damage to the immune system, can also develop naturally when certain diseases attack and damage the white cells of the body, but these are rare causes when compared with the frequent use today of immunosuppressive drugs for a host of applications other than transplant surgery. One of the commonest of these is the cortisone group of drugs which are widely used in medicine. These drugs do not by any means totally paralyse the immune system, but they do have very marked depressive effects upon it. The use of a cortisone cream, for example, will suppress anti-inflammatory action at the site of its application, usually the skin, and this will be helpful in many situations. Inflammation, though, is usually the outward sign of a battle by the body against an invader and in the case of a herpes infection a cortisone cream will of course not stop the virus growing, but it will slow down the body's response to it. In general cortisone preparations are not recommended for genital herpes for these reasons. This local use of cortisone is mentioned here, as this group of drugs is the most widely used of all applications to the skin today, and many people have a tube left over from some other occasion in their medicine cupboards.

The cortisone compounds are also very widely used by mouth in a range of dosages, so that their effects, as far as immune suppression goes, vary greatly in the individual taking them.

Should an attack of herpes develop in such a patient whose

immune defences are not working, or only poorly so, it will very probably be a severe one, as there is little to oppose the virus. The sores may be very numerous, large and widespread and take many weeks to heal, adding greatly to the patients' troubles, for, as we have seen, they are nearly always being treated for another illness or have had major surgery. The most serious complication to develop comes if the virus enters the blood stream. The disease may then spread round the body by this route, producing a very severe infection, which may be fatal.

Another and new example of immune suppression that we have briefly referred to earlier, which is naturally occurring, is the strange new illness which so far has affected mainly promiscuous male homosexuals in New York and California, known as the 'Gay Compromise' Syndrome, or simply as 'acquired immune depression' syndrome (AIDS).

Cases have also occurred in England and many other parts of the world and its cause is exciting much interest and investigation. The men who develop it badly have an immune system which appears to be totally and completely paralysed, so completely that no medicines could compete with it for efficacy. What makes the illness so serious is that the immune paralysis appears to persist for a long time and the results of this have been that many develop serious infections with a wide range of germs, some of which are rarely, if ever, seen in man. As some of these germs are difficult to treat with antibiotics and there is no help from the defenceless body, death ensues in a relatively large number of those infected. One of the illnesses which has turned up in this situation is, needless to say, herpes, and both perianal and genital herpes infections have been a serious problem in some of the patients. Finally, a variety of cancers have developed in other patients. Again it is assumed, almost surely correctly, that this is also due to failure of the immune system.

To find the cause of this mysterious illness would firstly save lives, but it might also give us some insight into how the immune mechanisms could be manipulated by the surgeon for his patient's benefit – in short we would like to know how, in this illness, the immune system is so completely and effectively paralysed and if it is reversible.

Before the development of the anti-herpes remedies cytarabine and vidarabine (see p.69), in the case of a transplant patient suffering from a severe herpes infection a difficult choice had to be faced. If nothing was done the viral disease – herpes – might kill the patient. If, however, immunosuppressive treatment was halted to allow the body's defences to recover and attack the virus, they would also attack the transplanted organ, which greatly increases the risk of its rejection.

Acyclovir promises to be much more effective and less toxic than these drugs, and trials have shown it to be most successful in dealing with herpes in the severely immunosuppressed patient.

Sexual Function

We have briefly mentioned the fact that herpes infections can interfere with sexual function on several occasions elsewhere in this book. These mentions have dealt with the apparently obvious reasons for this, such as the pain, worry and anxiety which interfere with the act. We shall now try to make this a little more explicit.

To carry out normal sexual intercourse, both men and women have to go through a series of changes which prepare and ready the genital organs for this act. The process is known as the sexual response cycle and its most obvious result in the male is erection of the penis and in woman swelling of the inner lips of the vulva and the appearance of moisture in the vagina – 'lubricating' or 'getting wet'. Neither of these responses is under voluntary control – we cannot command our sexual organs to respond in the same way as we can will our elbows or knees to bend. Hence the most important place in sexual arousal is the mind, as it is from here that feelings of sexual desire originate.

Once these feelings of sexual desire are under way, messages pass to the blood vessels in the penis and in the wall of the vagina.

These messages cause the arteries, which carry blood around the body, to open up, and the veins, which drain blood back to the heart, to close. As a result, the penis, being basically a hollow organ, soon fills with blood and, being fastened to bone at one end, it erects. In women the increased blood flow to the vagina causes the walls of this organ to become literally 'stuffed' with blood, which has, amongst other results, the effect of forcing liquid through the lining cells into the vaginal passage. This liquid has a similar composition to sweat, and along with a little secretion from some glands is what is responsible for the lubrication which is an essential part of the preparation for the act of successful intercourse.

Now there is a big practical difference here between men and women. This is that the switch which switches men 'on' sexually is a very strong one which is always ready to operate and is extremely difficult to damage in any way, certainly in most young men. Nature presumably designed it in this way, for if the male is not able to pass his semen readily to a female, the very future of the species is at risk. So it is to the species' advantage to have an efficient system of sperm transfer which is readily put into action and does not often go wrong. To encourage the male in this activity, nature has also ensured that not only is it an action easy to perform, but that it is also extremely pleasurable. This is of course a vital element in the male's 'competent' sexual performance – he is anxious to perform, he finds it easy to perform and, above all, finds the performance pleasurable!

When one looks at the equivalent response in women the important differences are quite obvious. Anyone can tell if a man is responding sexually. In many cases it needs some experience and consideration to determine if a woman is. There is no simple, erect penis signalling the situation in an unambiguous fashion! Then a full, or indeed any, sexual response is not essential for the act of intercourse to take place in a female. It will almost certainly not be very pleasurable if the response is lacking, but it can nearly always take place. This can't happen in men, who are not able to have intercourse unless their sexual response cycle has been completed

– that is, unless they have an erection. Thus the act can take place in women without any particular pleasure resulting. The very opposite happens in the male – the act of ejaculation which results from nearly every act of sexual intercourse he engages in is always pleasurable. As a result of this simple 'constant reward' system, he will always regard the act in a pleasurable and positive light – a state of affairs which is supported by his hormones, which maintain him in a state of easily arousable sexuality throughout most of his life, but especially so in his earlier years.

In contrast, many acts of intercourse in women are not automatically rewarded by the same degree of pleasure as the male obtains. As a result the constant reward system does not operate to the same extent as in men and therefore the 'sex drive' in many normal women does not seem to match that of men. This is to some extent clearly dictated by the ebb and flow of sex hormones in women. Men have an almost completely regular pattern of sex hormones, the main change being that most men tend to be more easily aroused sexually in the mornings – if they are awake, that is! Some cynic has pointed out that biologically speaking one can say that orgasm is a biological necessity for men but a luxury for women. Without going into the sexual politics of such an overstatement, one can see the biological reasons behind the provision of a very robust mechanism for sexual arousal and function, especially in men.

The result of this state of affairs is that sexual dysfunction tends to be somewhat commoner and more easily generated in women, perhaps especially so during the early and middle years of sexual life. Later, men acquire their own extra problems.

Herpes infections of the genital area can influence these sexual responses in several ways in either sex, leading to their impairment and a varying degree of impairment of sexual performance.

In the female most of these dysfunctions in genital herpes begin with the sores causing pain on intercourse. This will, if continued for some time, soon lead to a much lessened sexual response, with of course an exactly matching diminution of the pleasure obtained from the act. This is usually followed by anxiety – she may fear that the act is going to be painful, that she is going to fail again or sometimes that sex will cause another attack of herpes or that she may actually infect her partner. Add to this very negative collection of thoughts the fact that intercourse takes place at the time of minimal sexual arousal in the woman's cycle, and the stage is set for a complete failure of the sexual responses. If this is followed by intercourse or attempts at intercourse, they are liable to be very uncomfortable and this result may 'condition' her to expect or fear the same thing happening next time. Such fears (as in the presence of repeated attacks of genital herpes) are quite enough to ensure their translation into fact. The stage is then set for the possible development of quite serious sexual dysfunction, which may lead eventually to frigidity. After all, if sex is painful, depressing and humiliating because of repeated failures, it is not surprising that the patient rapidly begins to lose interest in it. Initially this is a voluntary suppression of feelings, though if such feelings are kept suppressed for a long time it may become a way of life. So herpes in women can cause painful intercourse, initially based on organic disease, that is painful herpes sores, though later on this pain may result largely from a failure to respond sexually.

Herpes in the male may lead to painful sex, though this is not as troublesome or as frequent as it is in women and most men can cope easily with it. If, however, the man feels his sexuality is under threat for other reasons, if the relationship is under stress, then fear of pain or fear of infecting a partner may be sufficient in such a man to cause so much anxiety that it inhibits even the strong male 'switch' of sexual arousal and the response cycle does not take place. If it recurs on a number of occasions, the anxiety so generated may be so intense that varying degrees of impotence or inability to achieve and maintain an erection will develop.

None of these sexual dysfunctions is directly due to herpes damaging any vital part of the sexual machinery. The underlying cause is psychological, originally based on a very physical cause, the pain of herpes. The only time herpes damages any part of the sexual machinery sufficiently to stop it working is when the nerves to the penis are temporarily affected in some severe primary attacks (see Chapter 3), but this lasts for only a few days and has no enduring effect.

Many patients are worried by the phrase 'psychological cause', as they fear that the doctor using it believes that they are inventing the symptoms or that it denotes some mental weakness or loss of character. It means none of these things – it is simply a statement of how the body and mind work together in every individual. We have some control over both, but in many ways our bodies at many times 'run us'. In this particular instance we want our body to make love to our partner, but our body in fact cannot allow this to take place as a result of our own anxieties (which are present both at a conscious and an unconscious level, and the latter may, in some individuals, be the most important).

Cure is achieved by explanation and attention to the specific anxieties. A clear explanation will often deal with most of them. With the loss of these inhibiting worries, sexual response and function usually returns rapidly, though supervision, encouragement and the use of certain simple sexual techniques may well be needed in some couples.

CHAPTER 10
Questions and Answers

In this book many aspects of our problem – genital herpes – have been deliberately reconsidered on a number of occasions in different chapters in order to emphasize important points. In spite of this repetition, many readers may appreciate brief answers to those questions about herpes and its complications which seem to cause the most worry. These questions will furnish, in effect, a brief summary of the main content of this book.

What is Herpes?

Herpes is an extremely common and nearly always mild illness caused by the herpes simplex virus. The infection is seen in the mouth, the lips, occasionally the eye, and in the ano-genital region. At any infected site, the virus produces a crop of spots which rapidly turn into blisters which ulcerate, leaving painful sores. Usually the whole illness lasts only for about two weeks. It is spread by direct contact between patients – skin to skin. Thus lip herpes is often spread by kissing and genital herpes by sexual intercourse or oral sex. First attacks tend to be severer in young adults, while recurrences are much less severe and may last only a few days. In a few, the rate and persistence of recurrences may produce serious problems for some.

Most people who are infected, however, are unaware of the fact, as no illness is produced, though the body will generate antibodies which can be measured in the blood. It is estimated that 70 per cent of all mouth/lip infections fall into this category and about a half of all genital infections.

The herpes simplex virus exists in two closely related forms, type 1, which is commoner in the mouth area, and type 2, seen more frequently in genital infections. As a result of oro-genital sexual contacts the viruses may be found at either site.

Very rarely, and in special circumstances, the virus (like many germs) may cause serious, even life-threatening, illness.

Is Herpes a Venereal Disease?

In the United Kingdom a special Act of Parliament was passed in 1917, the Venereal Diseases Act, which specified only three illnesses as being venereal diseases in law. These were syphilis, gonorrhoea and 'soft sore' or chancroid.

The word 'venereal' comes from the Latin for sexual love and strictly speaking any illness that is habitually spread from person to person during sexual intercourse can be classified as a venereal or venereally acquired disease. If this strict definition is used, genital herpes is a venereal disease. Equally, many other illnesses, including the common cold (and certainly lip herpes), can be acquired as the result of sexual activity.

I think it unkind to use the word in relation to genital herpes and a number of other diseases caught as a result of sex, as it does nothing for the physician from the point of view of scientific accuracy in diagnosis and nothing for the patient except to upset, alarm and frighten him. The upset and fear he feels are the direct result of the serious effects that the true venereal diseases used to have eighty years ago when they were incurable, added to a feeling that anyone with such a disease must be immoral and a fairly nasty sort of character. The public has a very long memory about such facts, even if those that were true (for instance the incurability) are long out of date, while the association of venereal disease with 'immorality' is a judgement which has to be an individual one in each and every case. A man who catches gonorrhoea after visiting a prostitute may have behaved in an immoral fashion, but if he passes the disease to his wife it would be very illogical to say that because she has venereal disease she too is immoral.

Most patients have enough worries anyway with their herpes without being saddled with additional and quite unnecessary extra ones because someone, usually the doctor, makes an unkind choice of name. I often recall a sobbing nineteen-year-old girl with vulval herpes who had been told she had 'VD' by her doctor. She had never had genital intercourse, but oro-genital sex had taken place while her boyfriend had a healing lip sore. Her herpes was bad, but what made her cry was not the pain this caused, but what the illness had been called. So, if any doctors read this book, please don't call herpes a venereal disease, or rather don't tell your patients with herpes that you think it is.

What Do I Do If I Get Genital Herpes?

The first thing to do is to make sure of the diagnosis and visit either your doctor or a clinic for sexually transmitted diseases. If the illness has followed a casual sexual encounter by you or your partner, the clinic is the best place, as they will be able to confirm the diagnosis by culturing the virus and making sure no other infections are present in addition to herpes. 'Double' infections are not uncommon, so this is a very important point, especially for women, in whom such illnesses as gonorrhoea are usually without significant symptoms.

The clinic or your doctor will arrange treatment and will advise you not to have sexual relations with anyone while the sores are present. You should also be careful to wash your hands with soap after touching the sores.

You should always inform your partner of what has happened, though it is possible that nothing will be found if he or she is checked, as the virus can be shed on occasions without any signs. If a third party is involved, partners should be strongly advised to have a check at a clinic to exclude other disease. Finally, make

sure you know or learn a little about the disease so that the incident
does not get out of proportion!

When and How is Herpes Spread?

Herpes is spread by the virus coming in contact with the soft moist
'skin' lining the lips, genitals, gut or eyes, and known as mucous
membrane. The virus is able to enter these cells directly once
contact is made with them.

To gain entry elsewhere, which usually means via the skin, a
break or 'breach' is necessary to allow the virus to enter. The
tough, scaly, outer cells of the skin are actually dead and it is
only those lying deeper that can be infected. For this to take place,
a break in the outer layer of cells is almost certainly essential. This
break may be very small, and will be too small to be seen with the
eye.

Spread usually involves the skin or mucous membrane being in
direct contact with other skin or mucous membrane, and in genital
herpes this nearly always means sexual contact. This may be
genital–genital, or oro-genital contact.

Very rarely an individual may introduce virus from one part of
his body to another ('auto-inoculation'), and the eye may be
infected in this fashion from a genital lesion by inadvertent
genital–hand–eye contacts. In practice, these are rare.

Virus is always present when herpetic sores are present, so such
patients are potentially infectious. The amount of virus produced
will vary from lesion to lesion.

Herpes can also be spread in the absence of visible herpetic
sores, the virus appearing from time to time in the saliva or
genital secretion of anyone who has been infected with the
virus. The amounts of virus produced and the frequency of its
production again seems to vary greatly from patient to patient.
Infection by such silent or random shedding of virus occurs,
though it is not very common. Such a happening is far from
rare in clinical practice, but it is certainly not the rule for

this to happen. A practical approach is to regard all herpes sores as infections and to avoid intercourse while they are present.

Is Herpes Curable?

Not at the moment in the sense that we have drugs which will rid the body of the virus completely.

Treatment will become available, almost certainly by the time this book is published, which will take the 'sting' out of severe cases of the disease. This is the drug acyclovir, which can be used as a cream or taken by mouth. It is effective in acute and recurrent cases. Its drawback, at first, will be that it is going to be quite expensive. It has been tried and tested and the delay in its arrival on the chemist's shelves is due to the complex bureaucratic procedures now involved in marketing any new drugs. These have been set up to ensure high safety standards for the public.

It is an important drug, too, as it is the first effective drug acting against a virus which can be given by mouth. There will soon be many more, and one or a combination of such drugs may root out the virus from its hiding place in the ganglia and achieve total cure.

Does Herpes Recur?

The answer is 'yes', but not in everybody. Recurrence is common and estimates vary widely from 40 to 70 per cent. There is little doubt that recurrence is rather more frequent in genital infections due to type 2 virus strains.

The frequency of recurrence is also extremely variable. Some people may get a recurrent attack every year or so, while others will develop them at two-weekly intervals. Recurrences too may persist for many many years, though there is a distinct tendency for them to decrease both in severity and frequency as time passes in many people. By 'time passing' we are talking of periods of two or more years.

A variety of different factors will precipitate recurrences and they tend to be fairly constant for an individual. Trauma to the skin, such as shaving, or trauma to the genitals during sexual intercourse, can be a common and troublesome 'trigger'. Stress is also an extremely common and important factor in promoting recurrence in some.

The reason some people have recurrences may be that they have been born with very slight weakness in their body's defence mechanisms, which appears to make them less able to combat herpes infections, though they are able to deal with other infections quite normally.

Can Herpes Affect My Baby?

Herpes can affect a baby in two ways. Firstly, like many other acute illnesses, a primary attack of genital herpes occurring during the first few months of conception may lead to an abortion taking place, though this is very uncommon in herpes. Recurrent attacks will not damage the baby growing in the womb in any way.

The other way that herpes can affect the baby is if there are any herpes sores on the genitals just before or at birth. The infant may then come in contact with them as it moves through the birth canal, and the risk of infection is high in such circumstances. After birth the child can also be infected by anyone in contact with it who is suffering from herpes sores though, for obvious reasons, people with genital sores are unlikely to be responsible. The enthusiastic relation, who may not realize how infectious his lip sores are and who wishes to kiss the infant, is perhaps the biggest risk. Once more, remember that fortunately herpes infections in babies in Britain are rare.

Does Genital Herpes Cause Cancer?

The answer is almost certainly 'no', but there is a distinct association between infection with the virus and many cases of the disease. The meaning of this association is not yet clear and it is being actively investigated.

Hundreds of thousands of women are infected with herpes, though only a very few develop cancer of the cervix.

Of the patients who develop cancer of the cervix, a high percentage have evidence of herpes infection, though by no means all.

This form of cancer can be detected before it is fully developed by means of cervical or 'Pap' smears, and women who have had genital herpes are advised to have these tests at regular intervals.

In short, the risk of developing cancer of the cervix later, should you be infected with genital herpes, is almost certainly no different from that of a woman who has never had the disease. Certain factors *may* increase these risks, however, and promiscuous sexual behaviour by the woman (or her sexual partner) *may* be amongst these factors in some individuals.

The age at which herpes is caught and the presence of other genital infections together with hereditary factors may also be of importance in the causation of cervical cancer.

What Are the Risks of Silent or Random Shedding of Virus as Far as Infecting Partners Goes?

Partners can be infected with virus shed from one of the sites of herpes infection, whether that virus comes from sores or is shed without any signs or symptoms. Virus makes its way from the ganglia in the sensory nerves, where, we have learned, it lives. From time to time it appears at the surface roughly at the site of original infection. It appears to be most commonly found in the mouth and, when affecting the genitals, perhaps a little more frequently in women.

The amount of virus that is produced is often very small, probably present for only a short time, and very intermittently, though this varies widely amongst individuals. As a means of transmitting genital herpes it does not compare in effectiveness with the presence of herpes sores, which are responsible for the vast majority of cases. In a patient with genital herpes, sores and virus may easily be continuously present for many days and thus the patient will be infectious for that entire period of time. The random shedding of virus seems to be for short periods – a day or perhaps even less. Also, the 'dose' of virus is undoubtedly small in this situation and we have seen that this is often an important factor in infection.

Asymptomatic virus shedding can often be the explanation why genital herpes occasionally suddenly appears in one partner of a couple who may have been faithfully married for a number of years. The explanation is that one partner was infected with herpes years ago, either with or without symptoms of the virus's presence. All their marital sexual encounters have taken place at a time when no virus was being shed, until one day, by bad luck, sufficient virus to infect the partner is shed during one of these encounters and an attack of herpes results. The virus has finally succeeded in its aim of moving on!

This is a very rare happening, and in practice the only thing to worry about is the necessity to avoid sexual contact when sores are present.

Finally, note should be taken of the tendency for viral secretion or shedding to occur at less and less frequent intervals after primary infection.

Does Herpes Ever Cause Cancer of the Lip or Penis?

In view of the association of herpes with cervical cancer, many investigators have looked at both these possibilities and the answer seems to be 'no'. We have mentioned a rather tenuous connection in that some evidence has been produced that a few of the partners of women with cancer of the cervix do develop penile cancer, but there is not even really a tendency, let alone a strong one, for the two to be connected.

Similarly, in lip or mouth cancers, there is no convincing relationship that can be demonstrated and, as we have seen, virtually everyone eventually plays host to the virus while only a few develop mouth cancer.

More about Penguins
and Pelicans

For further information about books available from Penguins please write to Dept EP, Penguin Books Ltd, Harmondsworth, Middlesex UB7 0DA.

In the U.S.A.: For a complete list of books available from Penguins in the United States write to Dept DG, Penguin Books, 299 Murray Hill Parkway, East Rutherford, New Jersey 07073.

In Canada: For a complete list of books available from Penguins in Canada write to Penguin Books Canada Ltd, 2801 John Street, Markham, Ontario L3R 1B4.

In Australia: For a complete list of books available from Penguins in Australia write to the Marketing Department, Penguin Books Australia Ltd, P.O. Box 257, Ringwood, Victoria 3134.

In New Zealand: For a complete list of books available from Penguins in New Zealand write to the Marketing Department, Penguin Books (N.Z.) Ltd, P.O. Box 4019, Auckland 10.

Also published in Penguins

THE F-PLAN
Audrey Eyton

The book that started the diet revolution of the decade, *The F-Plan* is, quite simply, a phenomenon!

Here Britain's top diet-expert, Audrey Eyton, reveals her exciting F-Plan diet, which uses fibre-rich foods to ease away those surplus pounds with a speed and permanence that will amaze you. Here are recipes, menus and remarkable health revelations – everything you need to know to make that slim, fit future realistically possible.

Penguin also publish an indispensable companion to this diet, *The F-Plan Calorie Counter*.

And, coming soon in Penguins

JANE FONDA'S WORKOUT BOOK

A bestseller from Iceland to Yugoslavia, this is Jane Fonda's extraordinarily successful programme of exercises and advice on diet for today's fitness seeker – *the* book that will help you help yourself to better looks, superb fitness and a more fulfilling lifestyle. Her programme is specially designed to

* burn calories
* improve the shape of the body
* strengthen the heart and lungs
* build up muscle stamina and flexibility

'You can't do better than follow Jane Fonda's example' – *Woman's Journal*

'Energy and enthusiasm . . . and the intimacy of one woman talking to another' – *Time Out*

Penguins on Health and Medicine

WELL BEING

We over-indulge in eating and drinking, consuming the wrong
kind of food in our diet; we exercise too little – or too much!; we
allow the intense pressures of work and family to overwhelm us; in
short, we do our best to destroy and abuse our bodies.

Based on the television series with the advice and support of the
Royal College of General Practitioners. *Well Being* explores how
we can take sensible and informed measures to look after
ourselves. From diet and exercise, the hazards of drugs, smoking
and alcohol, the diseases of modern civilization, pregnancy and
childbirth, to the state of medicine today and alternative methods
available, the emphasis is on encouraging us to take control of our
health, fitness and well being.

TREAT YOURSELF TO SEX
A Guide to Good Loving
Paul Brown and Carolyn Faulder

Basic, readable, sympathetic, this handbook deals with a range of
sexual problems that are more common than generally supposed,
and gives a series of exercises, 'sex-pieces', worked out after
extensive research, which, if followed honestly and carefully, will
help provide workable solutions.

'By carefully following them (sex-pieces), people can learn to
understand their own sexuality, as well as their partner's, to their
mutual advantage and pleasure' – Marje Proops

'Elegantly written digest of current sexual counselling practice . . .
avoiding coyness and genteelism' – *Pulse*